ALSO BY KELLY STARRETT AND JULIET STARRETT

Deskbound: Standing Up to a Sitting World

ALSO BY KELLY STARRETT

Waterman 2.0: Optimized Movement for Lifelong,
Pain-Free Paddling and Surfing

Ready to Run: Unlocking Your Potential to Run Naturally

Becoming a Supple Leopard: The Ultimate Guide to Resolving Pain,
Preventing Injury, and Optimizing Athletic Performance

BUILT TO
MOVE

BUILT TO
MOVE

The Ten Essential Habits to Help You Move Freely and Live Fully

Kelly Starrett and **Juliet Starrett**

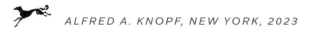

ALFRED A. KNOPF, NEW YORK, 2023

THIS IS A BORZOI BOOK
PUBLISHED BY ALFRED A. KNOPF

www.aaknopf.com

Library of Congress Cataloging-in-Publication Data
Names: Starrett, Kelly, author. | Starrett, Juliet, author.
Title: Built to move : the ten essential habits to help you move freely and live fully / Kelly Starrett and Juliet Starrett.
Description: First edition. | New York : Alfred A. Knopf, 2023. | "This is a Borzoi Book published by Alfred A. Knopf."
Identifiers: LCCN 2022008721 (print) | LCCN 2022008722 (ebook) | ISBN 9780593534809 (hardcover) | ISBN 9780593534816 (ebook)
Subjects: LCSH: Exercise. | Self-care, Health. | Movement education.
Classification: LCC RA781.S734 2023 (print) | LCC RA781 (ebook) | DDC 613.7/1—dc23/eng/20220701
LC record available at https://lccn.loc.gov/2022008721
LC ebook record available at https://lccn.loc.gov/2022008722

Illustrations by Josh McKible
Jacket design and illustration by Tyler Comrie

Manufactured in the United States of America

1st Printing

For Georgia and Caroline

I move, therefore I am.

—HARUKI MURAKAMI

CONTENTS

BUILT TO
MOVE

INTRODUCTION

Health is the ability to realize our avowed and unavowed dreams.

—MOSHÉ FELDENKRAIS

T HE YEAR WAS 2000, the place was Chile, and we were there to compete in the World Rafting Championships on the Futaleufú River. Although we'd never met before, both of us had been professional river paddlers for some time, an esoteric career choice in the United States, but not unusual in other countries. While rafting is the most fringe sport you can imagine here, in Eastern Europe, Australia, New Zealand, and Japan, it's a thing. Teams in some countries are even funded by their government.

That year, the U.S. women's team was made up of very accomplished competitors, longtime champs, a few of them whitewater legends. The men's team was a little more ragtag, a bunch of adrenaline junkies who'd discovered they could make some money risking their lives running Class V rapids—long, complex, violent channels of water.

We first laid eyes on each other when both the men's and the women's crews went down to the river to take a first training run. It was infatuation at first sight. In the Indigenous language Mapuche, Futaleufú means "Big River." To those local to the valley, it's referred to as *un paisaje pintado por Dios*—a landscape painted by God. The moment we met felt, well, biblical. Totally life-changing.

As the two groups prepared to get into rafts, we chatted and flirted in a way perhaps only a paddler could appreciate—and that proved prescient. Juliet tightened up Kelly's life jacket, while he loosened hers, a way of making fun of each other's safety "style." Juliet was wearing her life jacket tight because, like her teammates, she was pragmatic. (It's no accident that she has paddled her way to two world championships and five national titles.) If you fall into the water and your life jacket isn't snug, it's going to float above your head, which is not going to keep your body raised and therefore it won't help save you. But as for Kelly and the river guys, well, they had a tradition of keeping their life jackets loose, incautiously—maybe even brashly—choosing comfort over safety. Not a great idea.

The life jacket fiddling ended when both of our teams turned their attention to the business at hand: the roiling, cerulean waters of the Futaleufú. We each got into our boats and started down the river, heading toward the fabled Mundaca rapids. Mundaca is a gigantic chute of water, an elevator with lateral walls as tall as a school bus standing on end. It's a big, scary place even for seasoned rafters. As we got closer, the women's team pulled over to the riverbank, prudently studying the rapids before making an attempt. That's how you find the best and safest routes. What did the men's team do? The men's team headed straight into Mundaca. They thought they'd given this Chilean wall of whitewater enough of a look since we'd all scouted it earlier from about a half mile away. But that's like calling a strike from the bleacher seats. The information was useless.

Two seconds into Mundaca the men's raft flipped.

Class V rapids are not only high and fast-running troughs of water, they also have holes at the bottom that suck you down into liquid hell. So, when Kelly flipped, he was getting pounded, bounced, and squeezed into the depths of this big river—but not before watching his $400 paddle float downstream. Through it all he was—yes—trying to tighten up his life jacket in hopes that it would help lift him above the water. Then, suddenly, the women's team pulled up in their raft like superheroes descending upon a city under attack. That's when Juliet reached out a hand to a man she had only met a short time earlier, essentially saying, "Come with me if you want to live."

As meet-cute stories go, we think it's a pretty good one—and it should be noted that the women's team went on to take second place and totally saved the men's team's asses—but that's not why we just told it to you. What we learned that day in no uncertain terms is that you can't forgo the basics. No matter how many times you've gotten away with it, if you're not properly prepared, you may find yourself metaphorically (and perhaps even literally) up a Class V creek without a paddle.

Built to Move is our life jacket, handed to you, with instructions on how to prepare your body for whatever comes its way, be it aging, injury, or just the physical aches and pains that can come from living in this chairbound, technology-loving, caffeine-fueled world of ours. With this book as your guide, you'll stop "throwing" your back out when you make the bed. You'll no longer find yourself uncomfortably bent over when you get up from a chair after a long session at your desk. Your shoulders will relax. You'll lose weight and become less susceptible to related diseases like diabetes. Your spine will become more stable, your energy renewed, your mind clear. If you're an athlete or devoted exerciser, you'll be faster, stronger, and less prone to wrecking a shoulder or hamstring. Knee aches will fade. What you'll essentially be doing is building yourself one hell of a durable body. And you'll be doing it in some very unexpected ways.

To see what we mean, take off your shoes. That's right: shoes off. Now follow these instructions:

In an area free of debris, stand with one foot crossed in front of the other. Without holding on to anything (unless you feel very unsteady), bend your knees and lower yourself to the floor until you're sitting in a cross-legged position. Now, from the same cross-legged position, lean forward with your hands outstretched in front of you for balance, and rise off the floor—if possible, without placing your hands or knees on the floor or using anything else for support.

You have now just taken what's called the Sit-and-Rise Test. So, how'd you do? Don't worry if you didn't ace it. There's no public service message on TV telling you that you need to practice getting up and down off the floor. Doctors never mention it. Fitness trainers have other fish to fry. But being able to sit and rise without support is a singular way to tell if you've got a body that's dynamic and able to move in ways that will make you feel alive—and even help you stay alive longer. Same goes for hitting all the other usually overlooked benchmarks you'll encounter in this book.

The reason we hit you with the Sit-and-Rise Test so soon (we'll revisit it in full starting on page 30) is because we wanted to get you thinking about what being able to get up and down off the floor represents: mobility. "Mobility" is a kind of wonky term that refers to something quite beautiful: the harmonious convergence of all the elements that allow you to move freely and effortlessly through space and life. Everything is in sync— your joints, muscles, tendons, ligaments, fascia, nerves, brain, and the vasculature that runs through the body. The program in this book—and our life's work—addresses this whole network of movement components. Harnessing its power will help you achieve agility, ease, and quickness of step while vanquishing restriction, rigidity, and pain.

And, contrary to what you might expect, achieving good mobility doesn't call for exercise. No cardio. No strength training. Instead, it's a series of simple activities that enhance your capacity for free and easy movement, and in doing so also improve all the systems in your body (digestive, circulatory, immune, lymphatic) that are impacted by putting yourself in motion. You use your body's infrastructure, so you don't lose your body's infrastructure. Mobility also primes the body for exercise, if that's what you want to do. But more important, it primes the body for life.

The premise of *Built to Move* is simple: 10 tests + 10 physical practices = 10 ways to make your body work better. It introduces elements of well-being that most people have never heard of before, weaving them into a plan that everyone can accomplish in one form or another. Like the Sit-and-Rise activity you just did, the tests are markers of what we call

Vital Signs, indicators of how well you move, how much you move, or how well some of your other lifestyle activities support movement. You're about to find out things like whether you can raise your arms overhead without restriction, if you can balance on one leg, how high (or low) your daily micronutrient intake is, and how many hours of sleep you're getting per night. These aren't things that are traditionally known as Vital Signs, but we'd argue that it's just as important to gather information on these aspects of health as it is to chart your pulse, blood pressure, and cholesterol levels. These Vital Signs provide clues to why you may have aches, pains, and fatigue; they foretell whether you'll be able to recover well from illness or injury; and they serve as a harbinger of how active you'll be as you age.

This is info you can use because each test is paired with a physical practice—which can be anything from a series of mobilizations to a sleep or eating strategy or a combination of activities—that will help improve the Vital Sign in question. We've spun them all into a succinct, workable plan that anyone can do—and, we humbly suggest, everyone *must* do. We've been down in the fitness trenches long enough to learn that these are the ten things that matter, no matter who you are or how you spend your time. They are foundational. If you're a thirtysomething who wouldn't be caught dead in a gym and spend most of the day staring at a computer, they matter to you. If you're a triathlete, a CrossFitter, a retired golf enthusiast, or a midlife professional who only has time to hike with your dog on the weekends, they matter to you, too.

It may not seem like a twenty-three-year-old Olympic-caliber mountain biker who's been injured for the first time and a sixty-eight-year-old boomer grandma whose joints are creaky have anything in common, but they both need the same basic mobility maintenance—ways to address, preserve, and enhance the natural human physical condition. Maybe your goal is to swim across a rough ocean channel like a Navy SEAL or run the New York City Marathon. Maybe you just want to be able to get up from your desk after a marathon session of internet surfing without feeling a twinge in your back, or to roll around on the grass with your kids or grandkids. Either way, this book will help you. And trust us, it's going to feel good.

In health (as in life) people tend to get siloed according to various details—their ages, their activity levels, their abilities, their individual aches and pains. What *Built to Move* does is bridge that divide because, well, all bodies are built to move! Even if you're familiar with and regularly practice the advanced mobilization and movement techniques in Kelly's book *Becoming a Supple Leopard: The Ultimate Guide to Resolving Pain, Preventing Injury, and Optimizing Athletic Performance* (first published in 2011, updated in 2015), there's still a lot to be learned here. No matter what our extracurricular activities, as humans we're all fighting the good fight against gravity, technology creep, food confusion, stress, sleep disruption, and the inevitable process of aging.

What this book does is prepare you to play the long game. Throughout these pages, you'll read about some of the information we've gleaned from working with high-performance individuals. But as helpful and as interesting as those nuggets of wisdom can be, we're actually more interested in what's to be learned from the most durable people among us. Not what makes a star quarterback a star quarterback, but what makes the most durable regular people the most durable regular people. How is it, for instance, that an ordinary guy who is seventy-seven years old can go out, shovel snow in the morning, and spend the rest of the day sledding with his grandchildren, none the worse for wear? You've heard people edging into their fifties and sixties say, "Hey, I feel like I'm suddenly falling apart." What about people of the same age who are not falling apart? What makes them able to say, "Hey, I feel just as vibrant as I always have?" You'll find the answers to those questions among the ten Vital Signs we'll be introducing you to here.

When you're in your twenties, thirties, even your forties, it can be hard to appreciate the long game. You're not exactly thinking about whether you'll be at risk for falling or whether, as you get older, your lack of mobility will cause you to be a burden to the people who love you. But whatever age you are now, whether you skew into the lower "what-me-worry?" age group or are at an age where you *are* starting to be concerned about how you'll fare as the years advance, developing good movement health habits is going to pay off. And the best part is that you'll receive that payoff immediately, as well as later down the line.

In 2010, we created a company called MobilityWOD (Workout of the Day) and began posting a daily video on YouTube, focusing on, as the name suggests, mobility. It was a natural evolution for us because everything we'd been doing in the preceding years was telling us that using the body as nature intended it to be used—which few people, even professional athletes, were doing—was the key not only to better athletic performance but to better living. And we had a good vantage point: While we were both juggling family life and our day jobs, we began moonlighting in the fitness field, hosting CrossFit-style workouts in our San Francisco backyard, then eventually opening up a CrossFit affiliate in the city. It became plain to us that whether people were working their asses off at the gym and getting nowhere or showing up on Kelly's physical therapy table with intractable aches or injuries, a lack of understanding of how the body is supposed to move—combined with a lack of attention to basic mobility—was holding them back. Many had also developed unhealthy ways of coping with over-packed schedules, caffeinating by day to bring them up, using alcohol or sleep aids at night to bring them down. It wasn't long before we quit our other jobs and stepped away from the gym to focus on what the fitness world was overlooking: movement health.

When we started dropping those MobilityWOD videos back in 2010, we had no idea it would start a revolution. Before we knew it, "mobility" had become a buzzword among sports and fitness experts. As word traveled, we received calls from people all over the world wanting to learn more. Soon enough, MobilityWOD had morphed into our present company, The Ready State, and we were working on movement and mobility with all branches of the military; NFL, NBA, MLB, and NHL players and coaches; Olympic athletes; university sports teams; *Fortune* 500 companies; individual CEO types; and thousands of others.

But the thing about mobility that bears repeating is that it's not just what enables the physically elite or the well-connected to perform at the top of their game. It's what makes *everybody* perform at the top of their game—even if that game is *Minecraft* or *Fortnite* executed while nearly dormant in a chair. The practices that maximize mobility are the same for everyone. It turns out that what makes an elite athlete excel also makes a nonathlete a more agile, vital, and pain-free human being. And the great thing is, you hardly need to be an athlete to work mobility practices into your life.

Because, again, we're not talking about exercise. Exercise is vital for your heart and lungs, your muscles, your body composition, your peace of mind, and a hundred other things. As you might suspect, we're fans. We highly recommend regular exercise with no further stipulation other than that you do something you love (or at least like). It can be Pilates, paddling, running, swimming, Zumba, cycling, CrossFit, walking, yoga, powerlifting, whatever. We are totally agnostic regarding the best type of physical activity. And, as it relates to the subject at hand—mobility—exercise is extracurricular. (We'll have more to say about exercise on page 279.) None of those activities listed above replace practices that engage the muscles, tissues, bones, and joints in acts of simple yet vital movements. Nor can they substitute for the practices that support those movements. How much you sleep, for instance, affects how much pain you feel and therefore how much you move during the day. As you'll see going forward, it's all connected.

By now, you've probably gotten the message that being sedentary sets you up for all kinds of problems, dying prematurely being the worst of them. But somehow that message has been translated into the idea that if you pedal your heart out for an hour at SoulCycle or on your Peloton bike, you've conquered the sedentary dilemma. Props to you for working out, but it's not the same as moving your body throughout the day in all the healthy ways it's hardwired to move. Movement is putting your body in motion by way of stepping, bending, crouching, shifting your weight, reaching, pushing, pulling, even fidgeting. It's a combination of functional actions that keeps everything, joints to digestive system, in good working order. We all move in some way every day, yet most of us don't move enough or in all the ways we need to.

Indeed, from our brain on down, we are designed to move. And not always for the reasons you might think. It is well established that we are ambulatory because it allowed our ancestors to hunt and gather. Our sustenance relied on movement (and still does, if you count getting up from the couch and walking to the refrigerator). But other life-sustaining processes depend on movement, too. We need to walk because walking gets everything flowing in our body. It's how we nourish all our tissues, how we decongest, how we stimulate the body to release waste. We're also programmed to regularly come in contact with the ground. Early humans sat on the ground, slept on the ground, and toileted on the ground. In a lot of cultures, they still do, which may partially explain why they're able to stay more active in old age than your average American. It may also shed light on why people in the Western world are more likely to have joint pain and even joint replacements.

That doesn't mean we should all start eating dinner while squatting in front of the coffee table or give up our modern bathrooms. There's little sense in taking a romantic view of our Paleolithic selves—nothing dreamy about the days when you could die from something as simple as an abscessed tooth. Yet we could all use some of what, borrowing a term from conservation biology, we like to call *rewilding of the body*. Rewilding, in general terms, is defined as "restoring and protecting natural processes." Like any ecosystem, our bodies have an inherent design for optimal functioning. Everything in this book is geared toward reinstating that natural state of affairs. Rewilding.

It's clear that we need it. As is well documented, we are now a society that drives to the gym, has our groceries delivered, and logs more screen time than even Steve Jobs and Bill Gates in their wildest dreams could have imagined. We're not loading our bodies with the bone- and tissue-enriching weight those groceries might offer, and we are keeping our spines, shoulders, hips, and knees locked in unnatural positions for hours on end. Again, we are designed to move in certain ways. To do otherwise would be like taking an airplane for a spin on the freeway: Yes, it will drive in its own highway-inefficient way, but if you get it up into the air—the place it was built for—that flying machine will soar.

Seventy-three percent of adults in the United States are overweight, says the Centers for Disease Control and Prevention. Here's another big number: According to the Health Policy Institute at Georgetown University, 65 million Americans report a recent episode of back pain; some 16 million adults have chronic backaches. Now this: The Global Wellness Institute estimates that the fitness industry is an $868 billion business, and data shows we're exercising more than ever. That seems like a big disconnect. If so many people are shelling out money to gyms, yoga and cycling studios, running shoe manufacturers, and the like, why are we as a country overweight and in pain? We've become fatter, sicker, achier, less fit, are getting more joint replacement surgeries . . . the list goes on.

Part of this we blame on the messaging coming out of the fitness world. If you don't naturally take to physical activity or if you have physical limitations, fitness recommendations can be daunting. Plenty of people end up doing nothing because they jump into what they think they're supposed to do, unprepared for the exertion, only to hate it or get injured and quit. We're happy to report that fitness trainers around the country are now introducing the mobility drills we've popularized to their clients, helping to prepare their bodies for working out, something that makes it both easier and more enjoyable. Still, many of those who genuinely love exercise, and even elite athletes, still haven't gotten the message that there's more to being fit than a punishing session in the gym or on the road. If you want to see how good your fitness regimen is, runners go take a cycling class, swimmers jump into Pilates, yoga devotees try CrossFit—and vice versa—and see if you can move capably across platforms. If you're so hyperspecialized that you fall apart when we hand you a weight and ask you to do a lunge, you're not really that functional. And isn't that what we all really want to be? Functional at the level that allows us to do everything we want and need to do?

It's clear we need a different approach, and we think that approach is giving you the tools to perform basic movement health maintenance on yourself through a variety of practices that complement one another. This program is base camp. You can climb any peak once you've got base camp under your belt. Want to train for a 10K or a marathon? Cycle around a foreign country? Maybe your "peak" is regular weekend hikes or morning walks around the neighborhood. Regardless of what your goals are—it could be just fulfilling your daily obligations without being encumbered by a body that hurts—this is where you start for today *and* the future. The mobility you foster now will ease you into your later years as well as any 401(k).

Over the last decade, we've put tens of thousands of people through the protocols in this book and seen great results. And we don't just pay lip service to the ideas we're spouting; we do the ten physical practices ourselves. Because of the business we're in, we have access to every tool, every training plan, every piece of equipment, and every advanced fitness technology you could think of. We can call up the greatest, most famous athletes in the world and get advice. It's an embarrassment of riches. But what we do first are the practices in this book, and we do them every day. This is where we start and, frankly, when life gets chaotic—and it often does for two normal people with full-time jobs and two kids—these practices are all we get in. Sometimes it's all we can do to sit on the floor while we watch a movie (stay tuned to learn why this seemingly passive activity enhances mobility), eat three vegetables, and get a good night's sleep.

This is by way of saying that we're not perfect and we don't expect you to be, either. This ethos is built into our program. It's all very doable, you don't have to go to the gym, and there are a lot of different ways to do it, which we'll clue you in to in Making It All Work: 24-Hour Duty Cycle (page 267). We're not going to lie and tell you that you don't have to put some time into it (unfortunately, you can't just read the book and get all its benefits by osmosis!). Don't let anyone tell you that attaining good health doesn't take any effort. It does. But as two busy people who work these practices into their day, we can tell you that the time commitment is both reasonable and achievable—especially if you get your friends, family, and even segments of your community involved to add both accountability and camaraderie.

No matter what you do in life, this book is more about living consciously than trying to live up to impossible standards. Our goal is to get you to simply get out of a chair more often, take a few minutes to stand on one leg to improve your balance (what else are you going to do while you're brushing your teeth?), add roasted broccoli to your dinner plate, wear an eye mask to help you sleep. Walk. Sit on the floor while you watch TV. Better mobilize your hips, shoulders, spine. If you ditch these things for a while, just start them up again. Let them always be your foundation, your touchstone for lifelong well-being. And let them help you glide so easily through life that you feel as though you were built to move. Because you are!

TEN TAKEAWAYS FROM THIS BOOK

- An understanding of how range of motion and body position- ing relates to health, ease of movement, and the presence (and absence) of pain

- Measurable and repeatable diagnostics that will help you assess your current condition, where you need to go, and how you're going to get there

- Mobilization techniques for reducing stiffness and resolving pain

- Insight into how frequently you sit, stand, and walk—and why it matters

- Ideas for arranging your environment to foster healthy habits

- Strategies for better sleep

- Easy ways to get more micronutrients and protein into your diet, plus guidance on the things you think you need to eat but shouldn't

- Knowledge of how to use breathing to achieve better mobility, overall well-being, and stress relief

- A first aid kit for soft tissue problems. If something hurts, what do you do?

- Thorough knowledge of how to perform basic maintenance on yourself

- A skill set of practices that lead to better health and a more durable body

How to Use This Book

When we summarized the *Built to Move* program as "10 tests + 10 physical practices = 10 ways to make your body work better," we wouldn't blame you if you contemplated that tagline with both excitement and fear. Is there, after all, anyone who doesn't want a body that works better? No. Everyone wants a body that works better. And yet you may also be asking, Who has the bandwidth to incorporate ten new things into their life? *You.* You have the bandwidth to work ten new things into your life, and we're going to show you how.

First, though, we should make it clear that many of these ten things are really just adjustments to what you're already doing, not brand-new activities you have to shoehorn into your daily routine. You already sit, eat, sleep, stand, breathe, and walk; we're just going to show you how to change it up a bit. There will be some new things, too—mainly mobilizations—however, they're not onerous and can easily be worked into a busy schedule. And as we mentioned earlier, we're not going for perfection here: All we ask of ourselves is to do what we can, when we can, and we ask no more or less from you.

This book is focused on the body, but it begins with the mind. We want you to think differently about your daily habits, to look for opportunity for movement where you may have previously thought none existed, and to reconsider what it means to be fit. It's worth reiterating that you can work out like a fiend for an hour each morning, and healthy as that is for your cardiorespiratory system, it doesn't mean you can spend the rest of the day sitting in a chair and consider yourself in good health. The message that most of us have been hearing for years is that if you sweat really hard for a relatively prolonged time several times a week, it's enough to take care of your body. If you work out, the time and effort you put into it is not wasted—far from it—but the body also needs to move throughout the day. It benefits, too, when you sit less and stand more.

Then there's balance. Who but the elderly, afraid of the potentially devastating effects of falling, gives a thought to balance? But there's two reasons it's worth thinking about it at every age. One is Normal Accident Theory. This is a theory positing that in all complex systems, accidents will occur. We live in a complex world where pavement gets slick, bikes hit bumps, spouses leave their shoes lying in the middle of the floor. In other words, you don't have to be of a certain age to run the risk of falling. And we're all moving toward being people "of a certain age," if we aren't already. Working on balance and other aspects of mobility is like putting money in the bank so you can handle whatever comes up in the future.

And deal with what's happening now. If you have pain or particular limitations, the mobilizations we'll be introducing you to can help solve a number of different issues. Do they address every possible orthopedic and soft tissue issue? That would be encyclopedic material well beyond the scope of this book. But that encyclopedic material does exist! If you don't find your issue tackled here, we encourage you to go to our website, thereadystate.com.

Finally, a word about the tests. One thing to remember is that our bodies are dynamic. Depending on what you're doing day to day, your range of motion may change. All the tests in this book are diagnostic tools that let you take stock and tell you where you need to focus your attention. That's it. They're not value statements. So many things could be going on. Family stress. Work commitments. Overtraining if you're an athlete. There are a lot of variables. Your range of motion, your sleep and eating habits, how you breathe—they're all like individual credit scores. They're constant, then the next thing you know they're dynamic. You only own them today, and tomorrow you may need to do something to adjust them. Having these movement Vital Signs as your go-to monitor—like getting a physical, only more often and with no sitting in the waiting room—can help you understand what adjustments you need to make. And once you have that aha moment, easy fixes come.

There are many ways to launch into this program. It should be noted that the Vital Signs are not listed in order of importance, but rather are sequenced in a way that experience tells us makes for a smooth entry into new behaviors. In truth, you can adopt them in any order you like, and all at once or in dribs and drabs. There will be some of you who will want to read through the whole book, taking each test, and adopting each physical practice as you go. By tomorrow you could have a whole new regimen. It's doable. But it's also not the only way to go. Depending on how you know yourself to deal with change, working them into your life gradually is not only acceptable, it may be more practical. Later in this book, we'll give you some different examples of how to incorporate the physical practices into your day (see page 267), but you can also just choose your own adventure. Let your own needs and interests be your guide to which practices you want to adopt first and at what pace you want to add in the others. You can also choose how you'd like to space mobilizations out during the day depending on your schedule.

It's possible that you may look at the lineup of ten physical practices and know that you've already got some of them covered. Maybe you already eat more than 800 grams of fruits and vegetables a day or get eight hours of sleep each night. Perhaps your stand-up desk has allowed you to avoid sitting most of the day. Take all the tests and you'll know where you're at and therefore where you need to go.

One caveat: Sailing through a test, particularly a mobility test, does not give you a free pass to just forget about a Vital Sign altogether. We know; that sounds stingy. But there's no getting around the fact that there's no skill or quality that doesn't require practice if it's to be maintained— although there will be instances where you may need to do less work than someone who is trying to build from the ground up. For instance, if you can already get into a deep squat and hold it for five breaths, you don't need to do the physical practices (Sit-Stands) designed to help you work up to deep squatting. But you still need to spend time in a deep squat a few times a week. The end goal is to weave all the physical practices you need into your life. There are no hard-and-fast rules on how to do that, so choose the way that's going to help you succeed.

And what is success? First and foremost, it's to feel noticeably better than you felt before you began engaging with the practices in this book. Second, it's getting to the place where every change you've adopted simply becomes routine, habits that you stick to without even thinking about it. And third, success is being able to say, years from now, "I'm still active and healthy because I moved my body often and in all the right ways." It's worth noting, too, that success can be achieved at any time. It's never too late to start—or, if need be, to start over.

You're going to learn a lot about yourself going forward as you test your Vital Signs and take mindful steps to improve them. And what you'll find is that you have more power than you even knew: the power to inoculate yourself against pain, the power to energize your performance in every endeavor you undertake, and the power to maintain a durable body and good health year after year after year.

A Few Things to Know

While it's our intention to stay away from as many fitness-geek words and phrases as possible, sometimes you just need to call something by its proper name, jargony as it may be. Here are some terms you'll find throughout the book and how we define them.

> **RANGE OF MOTION**—Look at one of your hands. Now flex your wrist so that the back of your hand moves toward the outside of your forearm. Now flex it the other way so that your palm moves toward the inside of your forearm. Those movements display your wrist's range of motion. Like the wrist, each joint in your body has the potential to move to the end of a given distance. Each joint can also extend and flex in different directions; some can even move in many directions.
>
> Having full range of motion means you can move your joints

completely every which way they can go. Nature has provided you with a very good range of motion, but neither modern activities of daily living nor most forms of exercise (especially if you're devoted to mainly one type of workout) give you much of an opportunity to employ it. On an average day, most of us only take our joints through a fraction of the movement spectrum, though we have the ability—and need—to do much more. Just as muscles that don't get worked lose their strength, joints that don't get moved in all directions lose their full range of motion. The old use-it-or-lose-it principle applies.

END RANGE—The farthest point in a joint's range of motion.

FLEXION AND EXTENSION—Body parts move in all different ways, but there are two fundamental movements that we'll be mentioning throughout this book. Flexion is a movement that closes the angle between body parts, like bending over. Extension is a movement that widens the angle between body parts, like straightening your elbow or pulling your leg behind you.

MOBILIZATIONS—The body adapts to the positions you put it in every day. If, for instance, you sit in a chair all day or spend a lot of time driving, your hips' range of motion will shrink and the joints will become stiff. Mobilizations are techniques designed to counter the effects of this type of mono-positioning and lack of movement. They're not strength-building exercises. Rather, the beauty of mobilizations is that they take your joints to different places, unstick compressed soft tissue (skin, nerves, muscles, and tendons), and ingrain new patterns of movement. They also engage the brain, letting it know that you can access positions safely so that it doesn't put on the brakes when you try to move in certain ways. Breathing and contracting and relaxing the muscles also figure into mobilizations, too. Because of this systems approach, mobilizations help address the tight muscles and joint limitations that cause pain and/or sap the body of its natural suppleness. Mobilizations sometimes call for tools (nothing too fancy—see below) yet are often as simple as lying on your back and raising your leg.

Many of the mobilizations in this book will likely look somewhat familiar to you if you've ever done any static stretching (the kind of stretching where you hang out in a position for a minute or so). But there's a difference between mobilizations and traditional stretches. Stretching is typically biased toward one system of the body's movement system—the muscles—and works through passive tension. Mobilizations, by contrast, target multiple aspects of the body above and beyond the muscles, including connective tissue, joints, and the nervous system. Stretching, therefore, only partially does the job of improving mobility; mobilizations take you much further. (See page 23 for more on stretching.)

CONTRACT/RELAX—Most of the mobilizations in this book call for a technique called "contract-and-relax." It involves contracting a muscle (tensing or tightening is another way to think of it), then relaxing it (letting go of the contraction). Generally, you contract for a few seconds, then relax for a few seconds, and keep repeating the action for the suggested time. This technique comes out of a physiotherapy practice called "proprioceptive neuromuscular facilitation" (PNF), and the idea behind it is to train your brain how to control a muscle in a given position.

When you're putting yourself in a position where a muscle and joint are at their end ranges—which you'll be doing in many of these mobilizations to restore range of motion—it has less power. Think of holding a heavy weight in your hand. It's harder to do when your arm is fully extended (this is the end range) than when your arm is bent. But sometimes you'll need to hold something in a fully extended position—think of carrying a pasta pot heavy with water as you move it from the sink to the stove. That's where this contract/relax conditioning comes in. It tells your brain that being in that position is okay and allows you to recruit the muscles you need to make it happen easily and safely. Contracting and relaxing can also be used to self-soothe and desensitize painful areas (see page 190).

ISOMETRICS—Exercises that involve contracting muscles without moving the joints. Squeezing your butt while you stand in line at the coffee place is an isometric.

LOADING—This mostly means exactly what you think it does: adding weight to increase the force on your body. Typically, you'll hear the term "loading" in relation to strength training: When you lift a dumbbell, that's loading. However, there are many other ways we load the body in life outside the gym. Carrying something heavy like groceries, a storage box, or a child is loading. Taking a walk while wearing a backpack with some books or cans in it (rucking—we'll talk more about it on page 123) is another good example of loading. When you add repetitions to something you usually do once, that's loading, too, even if you're not technically adding weight to your body. So, getting up and down off a chair ten times is loading. Adding speed is another form of loading. Walk or run fast, and you're loading. Walking up a hill or stairs is also loading.

The purpose of loading is to elicit a positive adaptation response. This is true for your muscles and surrounding tissues and it's also true for your bones. Bones need to be loaded in order to stimulate a process called "remodeling." Throughout our life, bone cells constantly break down and are replaced by new cells—that's remodeling, and it's essential for keeping the skeleton healthy. But the process depends on certain triggers, and loading is one of them.

SYSTEM SUPPORT—Mobility depends on a supporting system. Throwing every range-of-motion exercise at your body and walking 300,000 steps a day won't get you anywhere if your tissues aren't nourished by nutrients and rest and you can't breathe properly in position. We often get into the mindset that improving our ability to be active only depends on being more active. But there's no separating activity from what fuels it. Nutrition, sleep, and breathing are the foundational practices beneath the foundational practices.

We've Anticipated Your Questions

There are a few questions we've come to expect, so we thought we'd answer them right up front.

Do I still need to stretch?

Although we talked a little bit about stretching earlier, it's worth elaborating on since stretching has become such a ubiquitous fitness focal point. Ubiquitous meaning talked about a lot, but does anybody really do it? Our observation is no. Our other, related observation is that people tend to stick with things that work, but most people do not stick with stretching. Could that be because stretching doesn't work? Yes.

What stretching does is induce tension in a big muscle. Cross your feet, bend over your legs, and try to touch the floor and suddenly you feel tension in your hamstrings. That's stretching. Unfortunately, many people think they're supposed to stretch because doing so exacts change in the muscles; only it hardly ever does. If you sit on the floor and fold over your legs for a long time, maybe five minutes, you may make your hamstrings less stiff, but nobody holds a pose for five minutes. Fifteen to twenty seconds is more like it. In most circumstances, passively pulling on a muscle doesn't really achieve much, and it certainly doesn't improve range of motion. To do that, you have to get not just the muscles, but the fascia (connective tissue surrounding muscles), the joints, the nervous system, the brain, the breath involved.

That's the difference between mobilizations and stretches. When you do a mobilization—a move that allows your joints to go toward their end ranges in positions that you're built to assume—you're in effect saying to your body, "Look, I'm spending time here, I'm breathing, it's okay." It's exposure therapy, signaling your brain that using your body this way is safe. You're not just pulling on tissues and hoping that they change. You're looping your brain into the action, which is how real change occurs. When your brain and body become used to being in a position, you can safely move into it when you really need to—to take big strides as you race to an appointment, to chase a toddler, to sprint the last fifty yards of a triathlon, whatever it is that requires an extended range of motion.

There is nothing wrong with stretching. It doesn't do any harm, and sometimes it just feels really good to stretch. But as far as getting a lot of bang for your buck, stretching falls short because it doesn't address all the aspects of the movement system. Stretching is fine; go ahead and stretch if you like it. But if you want to have less pain, move more fluidly, and be better able to recover from physical stress—whether it's from hiking over grueling switchbacks or carrying the laundry up and down the stairs ten times in one day—mobilizations, not stretching, are your ticket to success.

What if a mobilization hurts?

Many people forgo exercise because they simply find it too uncomfortable. They don't like the labored inhales and exhales, the strain on the muscles, the post-workout soreness (though it should be said that some people thrive on all of the above). We don't consider mobilizations exercise in the typical sense of the word because they don't involve accelerated breathing or muscle stress of the type you'd get from doing calisthenics or weight training. Yet you may feel some discomfort when you do them (with or without tools) and even some post-mobilization muscle soreness. That doesn't mean you're doing them wrong, nor that you have to feel pain to gain. But the point of mobilizations is to take the body into positions that are otherwise neglected, to shake off the rust, so you may feel your body giving you some feedback. You shouldn't feel sharp jabs of pain; that's a red flag. But some discomfort and even some residual muscle soreness is fine.

That said, mobilizations can be done at different intensities, and you have control of the decibels. If you're using a tool like a ball or roller and your tissues are sensitive to pressure, congratulations: You've found an area that can be improved with mobilization. For big muscle groups, we like four to five minutes of mobilizing per side. Most people can tolerate much higher pressures on their hamstrings and glutes but find their quads and thighs to be much more sensitive. Some of the best athletic systems in the world, like the Chinese Olympic lifting team and Thai fighters, actually have people on staff to walk up and down on the athletes' quads. Mostly they complain that the pressure provided isn't enough! We mere mortals can up the intensity by pressing down harder. If you're in a flexed or extended position, you can ratchet it up by moving deeper into the pose. By the same token, you can do the reverse to back off the intensity. Do what feels right for you.

Consider, too, that it's okay to "freestyle." Once you have learned the basics of using tools on soft tissue (which you will in the soft tissue mobilizations throughout the book), you can be creative and use a ball or roller wherever your body is telling you you need it. Say, for instance, you are rolling on a high part of your hamstring and it's no problem. Then you move the roller down just two inches and you can't take a breath because it's so tender. Keep at it, gently but continuously, because that's good feedback from your body telling you you need some input there.

Remember: You should always be able to take a full breath while doing any kind of mobilization. Breathing is a great built-in "intensity gauge." Listen to your own body. That's the best gauge of all.

When is the best time to do mobilizations?

The short answer to this question is: whenever you can. It doesn't really matter when you work mobilizations into your day, as long as you're doing them. Different times work for different people, and we can say that from personal experience. Kelly generally does his mobilizations in the evening. He finds it's a good time because he can do them while watching TV and there is really nothing going on at that time that's going to disrupt him. As an added incentive, doing mobilizations with rollers or balls provides input to the parasympathetic nervous system, the system that induces relaxation. It's a good segue to sleep. Juliet, on the other hand, is a morning person who tacks mobilizations onto her a.m. workout time. She uses them as part of her cooldown. If you're the sort of person who gets up at 5 a.m. to meditate and journal (or just to have some peace and quiet before emails or your kids start bombarding you), first thing in the morning may be your jam.

Should you use mobilizations to warm up before exercise? If you have something particular you want to work on—say, you felt slow on your run the day before and think you can benefit from some hip extension mobility, or your crampy calves could do with some rolling—then, sure, go ahead. But your warmup time is probably better used getting hot and sweaty (more on warming up for exercise on page 201).

In the 24-Hour Duty Cycle and 21-Day Built to Move Challenge (page 267), we'll give you some specific templates for working all the physical practices in this book into your day. Mostly what you need to know now is that you can get by with doing about ten minutes of mobilizations every day. All the better if you can devote more time, but everyone has ten minutes, so no excuses. And just consider that 10 minutes a day is 70 minutes of input into your movement system a week, about 280 minutes a month, and 25,550 minutes a year. It aggregates to a really impressive amount of time you'll spend on caring for your body, but without taking much time out of your schedule at all.

Do I need to do each mobilization every day?

No. As you'll see when you get to the 21-Day Built to Move Challenge (page 267), you can spread out the mobilizations and mix them up as you see fit. We recommend doing at the very least one mobilization every day and hope you'll work up to much more than that. As with anything, you'll get out of it what you put into it.

A Few Things You'll Need

Some of the mobilizations in this book call for pieces of equipment. Most are simple and relatively inexpensive. If you don't have them, you can improvise with things you likely have around the house. Here's the lineup:

LACROSSE-SIZE BALL—Because they're firm, these balls sink into tissue and help "unglue" them. A tennis ball, while softer, will also do the trick.

FOAM ROLLER—These cylindrical tubes, often used for self-massage, can be purchased from any seller that hawks exercise equipment. Sub in a rolling pin if you don't have one around.

EXERCISE BAND—These elastic bands help you position your joints properly. You can also use any kind of strap, belt, towel, or T-shirt.

PVC PIPE OR BROOMSTICK—Whichever you use, it should be about three to four feet long.

Before You Begin

Between the two of us, we spent a lot of time in school, yet we've never tired of learning new things, particularly when it comes to information about staying well, staying durable, staying active. We see this book as an opportunity to impart to you some of what we've learned, but by far the most important—and most interesting—information to be gleaned here is greater knowledge of yourself. At its core, *Built to Move* is about self-discovery. Can you move in all the ways you need to? How well are you really eating? Are you truly getting enough sleep? What things can your body do that you didn't even know it was capable of? Are the real reasons you might feel pain the reasons you thought they were? By the end of this book, *you'll* be an open book, and we can't wait to hear what you find.

GETTING UP AND DOWN OFF THE FLOOR

ASSESSMENT
Sit-and-Rise Test

PHYSICAL PRACTICE
Floor-Sitting Positions and Mobilizations

C AN YOUR ABILITY to get up and down off the floor provide insight into how long you'll live? A group of Brazilian and American researchers thought that it might, so they endeavored to find out. In a joint study ultimately published in a 2014 issue of the *European Journal of Preventive Cardiology*, the researchers gave the Sit-and-Rise Test—the same one we previewed in the introduction to this book and which we're now going to ask you to take again—to 2,002 men and women, ages fifty-one to eighty. Then the scientists went about their business for six years until it was time to check back in and see how the sit-and-risers were doing.

In that six-year span, 179 (nearly 8 percent) of the study subjects had died. After crunching the numbers, the researchers were able to determine that, according to the study data, an inability to get up and down off the floor without assistance is associated with a greater risk of death. Conversely, the higher a subject scored on the test, the greater the improvement in their statistical likelihood of survival.

It's reasonable to think, "Well, sure, the people who died were probably pretty old and, since old people aren't so mobile, they probably fell, couldn't get up, then all kinds of bad things started to occur. I'm not old (or even if I'm 'old,' I'm not feeble!), so I don't need to worry about this happening to me." But that would be missing the point. The upshot of the Brazilian and American researchers' work is that people who do well on the test have greater mobility and that greater mobility may make them a) less likely to fall in the first place, and b) in better all-around health. What this means is that, whether or not you're worried about falling, the ability to easily sit and rise is a reflection of your well-being (and, truthfully, anyone can fall at any age, so don't discount the value of being able to get up). If you can move in all the ways that allow you to get up and down with little or no support, then your body is stable, supple, and efficient. That is, it has qualities that will help you avoid pain, feel more vibrant, and participate in all the activities you love to do. That is something people of all ages can aspire to.

What we love about the Sit-and-Rise Test, and the reason we use it in our own work, is that it makes the invisible visible. Every day you go through the habitual motions of your life, using your body in ways so ingrained that you don't need to think about them. But what is it that your body really can and can't do? In what areas can you improve? You don't know until you take a look. By assessing this Vital Sign, you're opening the door to self-knowledge and paving the way toward constructive change.

Assessment: Sit-and-Rise Test

The primary goal of this test is to determine whether you have good range of motion in your hips. It also gauges leg and core strength, as well as balance and coordination, attributes that help you get up and down from the floor without assistance. The combined power of these elements allows you to move smoothly and, when you need to, swiftly: If you've got to walk fast or run, quickly bend down to pick something up, hustle up some stairs, or dance at your sister's wedding, your body will feel freer and you'll be met with less resistance from stiff joints and muscles.

Before you go forward, keep a few things in mind. You get a gold star if you can both sit down and rise straight up from the cross-legged position without using any kind of assist. That shows you have basic, baseline hip flexibility. But it's also okay to use an assist. Place a hand (or two) on the ground, roll forward onto your knees to brace yourself, even grab on to the back of your couch. Just being able to get up is valuable. There's no disgrace in not doing well or even failing this test. Getting up off the floor is not something you do every day, so why should you expect to be good at it? But you will be. Once you have your score, we'll show you how to improve it. So take the test and see how you fare.

PREPARATION

Wear clothes that aren't restrictive and go barefoot. Choose a spot where the floor is clear of debris.

THE TEST

Stand next to a wall or steady piece of furniture if you think you will need help. From there, cross one foot in front of the other and sit down on the floor into a cross-legged position without holding on to anything (unless you feel very unsteady). Now, from the same cross-legged position, rise up off the floor, if possible, without placing your hands or knees on the floor or using anything else for support. Tip: Lean forward with your hands outstretched in front of you to keep your balance.

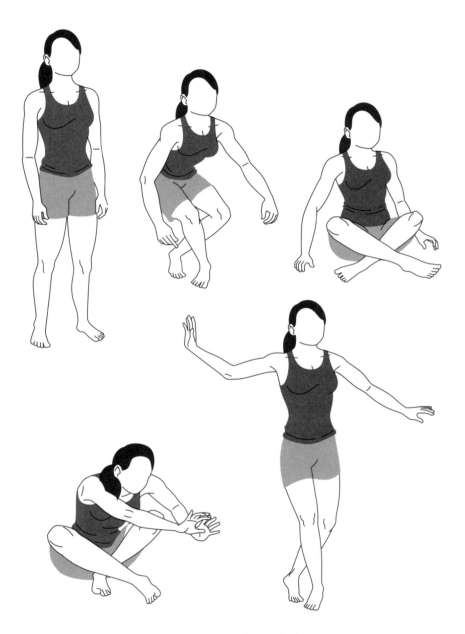

The Sit-and-Rise Test: It will get easier with practice!

WHAT YOUR RESULTS MEAN

Start by giving yourself a score of 10, then subtract one point for each of the following assists or problems:

Bracing yourself with a hand on the wall or other solid surface
Placing a hand on the ground
Touching your knee to the floor
Supporting yourself on the side of your legs
Losing your balance

Whether your score is good, bad, or ugly, think of it for what it is: simply a baseline number by which you can measure your prowess and then, if you need to improve (and almost everybody does), your progress. No matter your age or the shape you're in, strive to get a 10. Your ultimate goal should be to get up and down off the floor without using any points of contact, period. Does that mean you're a failure if you get below 10? No. Everyone, including us, will still like you. It just means that, while you get kudos for incrementally improving your score by adopting the physical practices we recommend, don't stop until you retest at a score of 10.

Also, no matter what your score, the prescription for improvement—or maintenance, as the case may be—is the same. That may seem like a bit of a bait and switch—higher scores typically mean less work—but the ground-sitting exercises and mobilizations that improve mobility are something you need to practice daily whether your goal is to improve or maintain. Again, the scores are simply there to help you gauge where you're at. Here's what they mean:

10 points—The gold standard. You obviously have a good range of motion in your hips and are blessed with other essentials of mobility. Don't, however, rest on your laurels. Do the physical practices to maintain your skill.

7–9 points—Congratulations, you're close. With just a little practice—it may be just a matter of attaining better balance or flexibility in the hips—you'll hit 10.

3–6 points—You're trending in the right direction but have a lot of room for improvement. Prioritize this physical practice, which will help you improve the hip range of motion you may be lacking.

0–2 points—Getting up and down from the floor is obviously very difficult, maybe even impossible, for you. Don't be discouraged. This is something you can master—and, with practice, you will. Rising without any support requires some leg and trunk control as well as balance and hip range of motion. These are things you can develop by habitually getting up and down from the floor and engaging in targeted mobilizations.

WHEN SHOULD YOU RETEST?

Every time you sit on the floor (ideally, every day), you can take the Sit-and-Rise Test again to see how you're improving.

The Beauty of Sitting on the Floor, or How (and Why) to Improve Your Sit-and-Rise Score

The Olympic Club in San Francisco is a refined, sports-centric private establishment that has been a fixture in the city since 1860. Its members can dine under chandeliers, golf on carefully manicured courses, and swim in an old-world, glass-domed natatorium. It's a pretty swanky place. So it wasn't all that surprising that we got some puzzled looks when we told all the members who'd come to hear a lecture on mobility to sit on the floor. Actually, they had no choice, because we'd cleared out all the chairs.

No doubt the attendees were expecting to hear about some kind of special stretches or unusual isometrics or some insider Navy SEAL mobility technique. What they got instead were instructions to make like a bunch of toddlers and position themselves crisscross applesauce on the carpet. We watched as they wriggled uncomfortably.

The point we were hoping to drive home at the Olympic Club that day is that sitting on the floor, if you do it regularly, is one of the things that can help you become more proficient at getting down on the floor, then getting back up again, without using any support. A related benefit is that it undoes some of the less effective (and sometimes pain-inducing) compensatory positions the body adopts after sitting in a chair (or on a couch or in a car; pick your body-always-at-a-right-angle poison) for hours at a time, day after day. Our bodies are built to sit in ground-based positions, so when you spend some time on your nice parquet floor or plush rug each day, you're helping to "rewild" your hip joints. Sitting on the floor restores their range of motion, which will not only make it easier to get up and down, but also potentially remedy the musculoskeletal issues associated with so much chair time. Let's break it down a little further.

CHAIR WARNING

Kids have no trouble sitting on the ground in all different kinds of positions for hours at a time. It's probably no accident, then, that they are equally adept at the related skill of getting back up again. This last action is so basic to the nature of childhood that we don't even notice that kids are doing it all the time. But when you closely observe toddlers, as a group of child development psychologists at New York University did in a 2012 study, it becomes clear just how easily—and frequently—kids pop up and down. The researchers found that twelve- to nineteen-month-olds fell an average of seventeen times per hour. These intrepid toddlers traveled over 2,000 steps within the same time frame, which means they also got up about seventeen times per hour. Luckily, we adults don't have to get up and down that often, but we could: We have the capabilities to both comfortably sit on the floor and easily get back up again.

Why have most of us lost these elementary abilities in the first place? It all comes down to one simple object: the chair. Sitting on chairs and other objects goes back at least 12,000 years, to the Neolithic era. The ancient Egyptians regularly used them; King Tut was even entombed with one. But as Galen Cranz reports in *The Chair: Rethinking Culture, Body, and Design*, some cultures firmly resisted the draw of what became so ubiquitous in Western culture, and still do. The right-angle seated position is embraced by only a third to a half of people in the world, writes Cranz, a professor in the architecture department at the University of California, Berkeley. People in non-Western countries, she points out, might squat to wait for the bus, kneel to eat, sit cross-legged to write a letter. This may account for why people in China, for instance, have 80 to 90 percent less occurrence of arthritic hip pain than Westerners. Using the hip joints as nature intended keeps them healthy and pain-free.

The cross-legged position, in particular, is beloved by non-Western cultures. The anthropologist Gordon Hewes, who conducted a worldwide survey of differing postural styles, noted that it is the predominant way of sitting in the areas of North Africa through the Middle East to India, Southeast Asia, and Indonesia, and many places in Central Asia, Korea, Japan, Micronesia, and Polynesia. Hewes's research goes back a while—to the late 1950s—but the cultural differences he found are still largely true today. According to Cranz, "One thing is certain: our [Western] chair habit was created, modified and nurtured, reformed and democratized in response to social—not genetic, anatomical, or even physiological—forces."

In other words, that tug you feel to sit in a chair as you wait for your number to come up at the DMV is more habitual than innate. We aren't meant to be molded into a chair shape all day long and, in fact, it's a very breakable habit. Once you start sitting on the floor and standing more (Vital Sign 9), you'll find that it not only feels natural but that you crave it.

To understand why sitting for long stretches fools with your physiology, here's a little anatomy lesson. We promise it won't get too complicated, but knowing a little bit about how your body works will help you better understand why we're asking you to do some things differently.

When you sit on a chair, you primarily rest the weight of your upper body on your hamstrings (the large muscles and connective tissue on the back of the leg that cross the knee and the hip) and your femurs (upper thigh bones). The femurs are connected to your pelvis, that big bony structure at the base of your spine, through the hip sockets. The tops of the femurs are like little balls, and they fit right into those sockets. The relationship between the femurs and the pelvis is important because it creates stability throughout your body. And stability is important because it allows your body to function at its best. Lack of a stable pelvis-leg relationship can lead to a host of issues like back and knee pain. Everyone needs stability.

The femur-pelvis stability-building relationship is something our bodies begin to develop early on in life. In fact, that's one reason we don't want babies to skip the crawling stage and just move right into walking (turns out early walking isn't a win in the my-kid-is-more-extraordinary-than-yours Olympics, after all). Crawling puts weight on the femurs in ways that set the hips up well for the future.

As an adult, you still really want your pelvis and femurs to be working together to create stability. But when you sit on a chair in the traditional right-angle fashion—and do so for the freakish amount of time that many of our lives demand—the femurs just end up resting in one position, and it's a position that isn't great for fostering stability.

What happens without that support? Your body solves the problem another way, usually by enlisting the long muscles in the back and in the legs to keep your body from moving in various directions. (We call those muscles the "four horsemen": psoas, iliacus, quadratus lumborum, and rectus femoris.) The efforts of those muscles take a toll when you've been sitting for a long time. They've tightened to keep you stable, and your brain has gotten used to directing them to do so. When you stand up, they stay engaged, tugging on your spine and creating discomfort. How many times has your back felt all rigor mortis and achy when you get up from a long bout of sitting in a chair?

Your knees may hurt, too. "Theater sign" is what physical therapists call knee pain caused by a long stretch of sitting in a chair. Your rectus femoris, which is one of the big hip flexors that crosses over the kneecap, gets stiff and tender from trying to hold you up.

Another casualty of prolonged sitting in a chair is that your bones don't get "loaded" in the proper way. If you remember from page 22, loading—putting weight on a body part—stimulates the normal, cyclical process of breaking down then rebuilding bone and muscle. There are weight-bearing surfaces in your pelvis called "ischial tuberosities," better known as the sit bones, which you often hear a lot about in yoga. In a chair, they don't get the burden they deserve. Instead, that weight rests on top of your femurs and hamstrings. Sit there for a long time and, particularly if you're a fairly big human being, that's a big squash of a panini on your hamstrings and other tissues in the vicinity. And it really mucks up the system. Fluids like lymph stagnate and the tissues—muscles, fascia, connective tissue—stop sliding and gliding, inhibiting smooth movement. It's like lying on one of those memory-foam mattresses. Those tissues, flattened by lack of lymph and blood flow, don't pop back up for a while, and that degrades mobility. All of which we'll get into later.

HOW TO MAKE CHAIR SITTING BETTER
FOR YOUR BODY

We're not saying you should never sit in a chair; that's not real life, especially at work. You will, we will, mostly everybody in the Western world will sit in a chair at some point during the day. So here are three tips for dealing with the inevitable.

1. Choosing a comfortable chair, of course, goes without saying. But, also, don't be fooled by the idea that a $1,000 desk chair that's advertised as having life-changing lumbar support will solve all your problems. This is for the simple reason that most people lean forward to type on their keyboards and don't even utilize the lumbar support. Sure, if you work by leaning back a lot, it may help. But be aware of your own working style before you shell out a lot of money for a fancy chair.

2. While we're on the topic of chair backs, consider that chair backs were once only for the privileged. Most people, if they sat on anything other than the floor, sat on a stool or bench, points out Harvard evolutionary biologist Daniel Lieberman in his book *Exercised*. This is still a good idea because, when you don't have a chair back to depend on, you turn on more musculature, build greater stability, and avoid the weakness that can lead to back pain. If you can choose a backless seat, go for it. Don't, however, make it a big balance ball, which is a popular desk chair replacement these days. Besides being only one height (see the tip below), you can't get stable on balance balls, whereas you need solid ground to create stability. Try standing on a mattress for ten minutes and you'll see how old this unsteady surface gets.

3. There's a sneaky way to get a more robust position in your chair by adjusting its height (this only works with chairs that have rollers at the base). Set the height of your chair higher than usual, then see if you can get enough purchase with your feet to scoot the chair back and forth. When your chair is set high, it's hard to powerfully move the chair, which is what you're going for. So now lower the chair an inch and repeat. Stop lowering when you reach the point where you can really use your legs to powerfully scoot back and forth; you'll be able to tell the difference from how it felt when you were sitting too high. Being able to put some power into your movements means that the placement of your feet and height of your hips are such that they'll support your spine as you sit.

WHEN YOU SIT ON THE FLOOR . . .

The bottom line is that sitting for hours and hours at a time inhibits healthy movement, no matter if you're on a chair or on the floor. But everyone sits at least some of the day, and by allotting some of that sitting time to floor sitting, you'll avoid many of the problems that slotting yourself into a chair for hours on end can cause. And, of course, you'll also train your body to get a 10 on the Sit-and-Rise Test.

When we talk about sitting on the floor, we're not just referring to sitting cross-legged. You can get benefits from sitting in all different kinds of positions. Kneeling, for instance. And squatting, something we'll talk more about in Vital Sign 7. These are all positions that allow you to organize your body in ways that lessen the force on the spine and enable you to breathe fully. There's a reason that cross-legged sitting and kneeling are the postures of choice for meditation, the former most especially. As you butterfly your legs out, you rotate the femurs in the hip capsule—this is called externally rotating the hips to their end range—and create a very stable platform upon which to sit. If you need to sit for any length of time as you're encouraged to do in meditation, this is the way to do it. It's kind of the difference between balancing your upper body on the head of a pin versus setting it atop a four-by-four-foot board. One is obviously going to keep you steadier. And whereas chair sitting downregulates the femur-pelvis relationship, cross-legged sitting resets the relationship.

Our goal is not to train you to be like Buddhist monks who can meditate for four hours in the cross-legged position. You don't have to always sit that way, or even sit that way for a long period of time (again, we discourage parking yourself in any seated position for endurance intervals). Being on the ground in other positions also provides some of the same payoffs, including loading up the bones, joints, and tissues in ways that keep them in their best working order.

Here's the other thing about sitting on the floor: What goes down must come up. Remember all those babies getting up off the floor seventeen times an hour? It would be great if we all got up off the floor throughout our lives—not as frequently as toddlers, of course, but at least once or twice a day.

Physical Practice: Floor-Sitting Positions and Mobilizations

While we've just extolled the virtues of floor sitting, it's not the only way to get better at sitting and rising. Doing a few targeted mobilizations will also help. Both floor sitting and mobilizations improve mobility by working on hip flexion, the forward movement of the hip joint (you'll be working on its opposite, hip extension, in Vital Sign 3). Doing both physical practices every day will give you the best results.

The floor-sitting exercises may seem very familiar to you, but we doubt that any gym teacher, fitness trainer, or workout book has recommended them as a means of improving your well-being or performance. That's probably why few people in the Western world, outside of floor-sitting preschoolers, engage in them. Just to show you how infrequently they're practiced, some of the Olympic Club crowd—a group that was pretty athletic—actually had to lie down because they couldn't sit cross-legged or on their knees or sidesaddle. Most adults (other than parents of toddlers) simply don't place themselves in these positions, even though they are fundamentally human ways to arrange the body. So don't be concerned if you can't master all the positions. Practice will help, but the fact that there are a few different options will also give you some latitude. Do what you can do until you can do more.

Finally, before you launch into these practices, remember that they do more than just help you improve your sit-and-rise capability. All the positions they put your body into help build stability and agility and take the pressure off muscles and other tissues that get stressed by repetitive patterns. Do these daily and you're simply going to be looser, experience less pain, and feel better all the way around.

FLOOR-SITTING POSITIONS

Sitting on the floor in a few different shapes is all that's required of you here. You can lean lightly against the back of a couch or a chair or against a wall for support (ideally working toward moving away from any props), and you don't have to stay in one position on the floor. Earlier we talked a lot about cross-legged sitting. Crisscross applesauce does a fine job of rotating your hips in ways that sitting in a chair does not. But other positions also benefit range of motion and thus mobility. Sitting in the 90/90 position (page 44), for instance, rotates the hip two different ways. When you're in the Long Sitting position (page 44), you fire up what we call the "posterior chain"—the hamstring, glutes, and calves, muscles that are the movement engines of the body.

Having a variety of positions to move into also allows you to fidget. Fidgeting is a good thing. It's your brain telling your body, "Get out of that position." Sitting in a chair really isn't conducive to fidgeting because chairs are so constraining. Just think of the La-Z-Boy. You can sit in a La-Z-Boy almost without moving at all. It's designed that way! We want you to fidget and change positions while on the floor because it gives you the opportunity to rotate your hips into different end ranges, take pressure off your tissues, and avoid stiffness and pain. Your brain is going to tell you to move around while you're on the floor, and that's exactly what we think you should be doing.

Your ultimate goal here is to work up to sitting on the floor at least thirty *cumulative* minutes a day, every day. Start where you're at and work up to thirty. Again, use the back of a couch or a chair or a wall for support if you need to. If five minutes feels like all you can do, there's your starting point. Begin with five minutes in position 1. When you're able to add five minutes more, include position 2. Work up to sitting in all four positions described below, staying in each for as long as comfortable and switching back to others if that feels right. You can spend all thirty minutes sitting on the floor while watching TV, or break it up. Spend ten minutes sitting on the floor while you work on your laptop (there are plenty of adjustable standing desks, floor desks, and low tables on the market that will allow you to work while crisscross applesauce), another ten as you talk on the phone, a final ten while you sip a cup of tea. We like to take a half hour out of the time we spend bingeing the latest must-see show and sit on the floor. We make our kids do it, too.

1. Cross-Legged Sitting

With your butt on the ground, bend both legs and cross one in front of the other, your heels tucked under your legs. Try to sit with your back straight or with your torso leaning slightly forward. Occasionally switch legs so that both legs take a turn in the front.

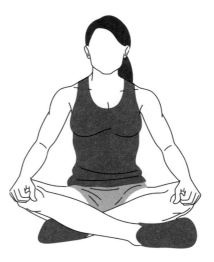

Cross-Legged Sitting maintains and restores hip and low back function.

2. 90/90 Sitting

With your butt on the ground, sit with one leg at a 90-degree angle in front of you (your thigh will be straight out from your hip). Slightly resting on the front leg's side of your butt, bend the other leg at a 90-degree angle so that its foot is behind you. After five minutes (or however long is comfortable) in this position, switch sides.

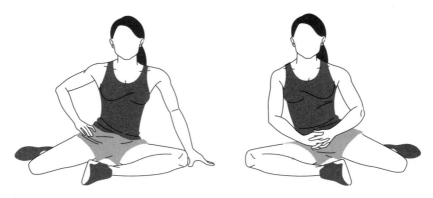

The 90/90 Sitting is an easy way to maintain movement capacity and movement options.

3. Long Sitting

With your butt on the ground, sit with your legs straight in front of you. Try to sit with your back straight or with your torso leaning slightly forward.

Adding Long Sitting to your floor routine keeps those hamstrings and calf tissues supple.

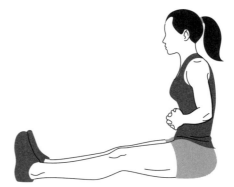

4. One-Leg-Up Sitting

With your butt on the ground, sit with your legs straight in front of you. Bend one leg, keeping its foot flat on the floor. Clasp your hands around the bent leg for stability. After five minutes (or however long is comfortable) in this position, switch sides.

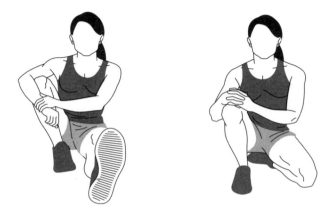

Get creative and get comfortable. There are no wrong ways to sit on the ground. Variety is the goal.

MOBILIZATIONS

These mobilizations not only go hand in hand with the floor-sitting positions in terms of boosting your sit-and-rise ability; they make the floor-sitting positions easier by training your body to stay longer and get up more easily. They do other things as well. The Seated Hamstring Mobilization feels like a self-massage, but what it's actually doing is loosening up the tissues in the backs of the legs so they move more fluidly. Other mobilizations help the brain learn to control movement. Collectively, they'll help you score that 10 on the Sit-and-Rise Test.

Think of these mobilizations as little microdoses of movement. They're simple; you don't need a super sophisticated intervention to increase mobility. You just need to start reintroducing your body to these very natural movements. There are four mobilizations in all. The ideal is to do two of them every couple of days (even if you passed the Sit-and-Rise Test). You can choose which two, but you'll have the best results if you alternate them.

You'll need a little bit of equipment for these exercises:

A lacrosse, tennis, or other similarly sized ball
A strap, flexible belt, rope, or exercise band

1. Seated Hamstring Mobilization

This action will help restore the sliding surfaces of the muscles and other tissues that lose function from too much sitting.

Sit on a chair or bench or tabletop—anything with a hard surface that allows you to have one leg straight out in front of you and one leg to the side. Place a ball or roller underneath your front-facing leg just below your butt, then extend the leg. Contract and straighten your leg, then alternately relax and bend your knee as you shift side to side on the ball or roller, using a sawing motion. Keep repeating the motion, working the ball or roller down your leg from your hip toward your knee as you go, about two minutes or as long as five minutes on each side.

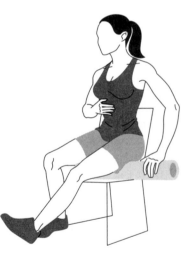

Mobilizing while seated is one of our favorite ways to sneak in some soft tissue mobilization.

2. Hamstring Lockouts

By contracting and relaxing the leg muscles in this position, you teach the quadriceps (the large muscles in the front of the thigh) to work against the stiffness in the hamstrings. This mobilization is also a sneaky way to get you to spend two minutes (per side) at the end of your range of motion. If you don't have a strap or band, a belt or piece of rope will do.

Lie on the floor, a strap or band at your side. Raise one leg at as close to a 90-degree angle as possible and wrap the strap around the arch of your raised foot. Tighten (flex) your thigh so your leg is as straight as you can get it and pull your foot toward your head. Don't force it; you just want to feel some tension. Relax your thigh, then tighten it again and pull your foot toward your head. Repeat tightening and relaxing for two minutes or until you reach four or five minutes. Switch sides. Try to keep tension on your hamstrings when you relax your quads.

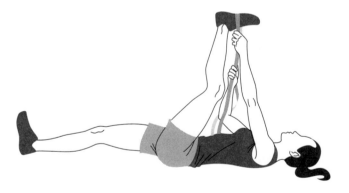

Lockouts are a staple with every population we work with,
from professional athletes to our own children.

3. Hip Opener

A mobilization for improving hip flexion, hip extension, and overall hip function, it lets you get into those tight corners of the hips.

Get down on the floor, then extend your left leg behind you and place your right leg in front of you, knee bent, shin vertical, foot flat on the floor. Try to take some big breaths here. Move your right knee around as if you're following the "rays" of the sun's 360 degrees, moving it forward along the line of one ray, back to the center, then along the line of the next ray over, and so on until you've completed a revolution. Use these movements to find out where you feel restricted, then work that tight area a little more. See if you can't collect two to three minutes noodling around before you switch legs. Take as many breaks as you need.

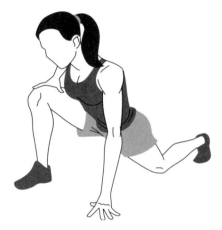

This is a sneaky way to expose your body to more full-range hip movement in a safe and controlled manner.

4. Elevated Pigeon

In this position, you're exaggerating the same hip position you use to sit cross-legged. It's similar to the pigeon pose used in yoga, but the setup is much easier.

Place your right foot on the left side of a bench (or tabletop), letting your knee drop to the side and your calf lie across the bench so it's perpendicular to your body. Sprawl your left leg behind you. Place your left hand on your right foot, "stapling" the foot to the bench, and place your right hand on your right knee for stability. Lock your arms and keep your shoulders back. Rotate toward your left side, then rotate toward your right side. Continue alternating between the two positions for two minutes to five minutes a side. Switch sides. You can always place a pillow under the knee of the leg you are working or drop your foot off the edge of the table to make this more comfortable.

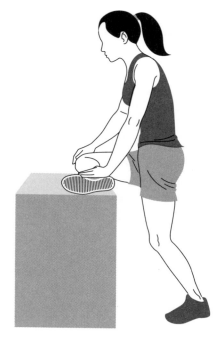

There is a reason pigeon pose is a staple in many movement traditions.

CAN'T I JUST DO YOGA? HOW ABOUT PILATES?

In a word, the answer to these questions is no. Yoga, Pilates, tai chi, qigong—they are all fantastic, but they are *movement* practices. They are ways to practice moving, not ways to restore range of motion. It's true that all these movement practices include positions that are advantageous to range of motion. The Indians who developed the physical system of yoga knew what they were doing when they created poses that prime the body to sit cross-legged, which itself (as you are learning in this chapter) takes the hip joints to their end range. Yoga, tai chi, and qigong also allow you to practice balance and breathing through the nose, other components of good mobility. All these traditional movement practices are practiced barefoot, too, which has its own rewards: The feet provide rich sensory input to the brain, helping you attain awareness of your position and use the rest of your body accordingly. Some people even theorize that the reason there's so much back pain in the world is because our feet are deprived of sensation.

If you are a devotee of yoga or any other movement practice, you will definitely get something out of it. These practices were designed to solve physical problems—Joseph Pilates was a genius at it. Yet they are incomplete. They are not like this program, a base camp program, a series of systems designed specifically to improve mobility and overall health. Yoga and Pilates, like other forms of exercise, are extracurricular practices; they don't make up for hours of inactivity the remainder of the day. They aren't compensation for sitting all the time, not sleeping, not walking enough. The takeaway here is the same as what we tell our running athletes, cycling athletes, and weightlifting athletes: You need the fundamentals to get better at your chosen activity and to fill in the blanks that they don't cover.

One thing we've found with yoga practitioners in particular is that they assume yoga has them covered on all fronts. When it comes to your health, yoga is not a cure-all for every physical dilemma (nor is anything else, for that matter). And we want to be sure to point out—because this is a common misconception—that yoga doesn't build muscle to any significant degree. Building strength, on the other hand, can help you be better at yoga. So, too, can improving your range of motion through the ten physical practices in this book. That's going to give you better access to the positions practiced in yoga.

BREATHE EASY

ASSESSMENT
Breath-Hold Test

PHYSICAL PRACTICE
Breathing Exercises

BREATHING IS NOTHING new; we've always done it. What we mean by that is, people—from disciples of the fifth-century yoga texts to Native Americans living on the plains to followers of the 1970s breathwork (and LSD) pioneer Stanislav Grof, MD—have been using conscious breathing for good health, psychological quietude, and spiritual contentment throughout history. And breathing seems to be having a moment again right now, with hordes of books on the subject, swathes of breathwork classes and breathing apps on offer, and even watches that—*ding!*—remind you to inhale and exhale on cue.

We're enthusiastic about all of it. Anything that promotes the idea that—far from just being the automatic response that keeps your heart beating—breathing is a tool you can use to control everything from blood pressure and immunity to anxiety levels gets a thumbs-up from us. But we also have a take on the benefits of breathwork that is often obscured by the chatter about its mind-calming and cortisol-lowering effects: How well you breathe has a direct correlation to your body mechanics, helping you move more efficiently, avoid injury, and feel less musculoskel-etal pain. In fact, when people come to us with persistent back and neck aches, the first thing we look at is how they're breathing.

So, what does it mean to breathe "well"? As we define it, breathing well boils down to three fundamentals:

Breathing *spaciously,* meaning that your belly, ribs, and chest expand generously as you inhale. These body parts are built to move as you breathe, not just to maximize oxygen intake, but also to allow you to take in enough air to help pump out waste-carrying fluid from your trunk and to create a sort of pressurized chamber that provides stability for your spine. (That's one reason breathing well can help you avoid back pain.) Breathing is initiated by the diaphragm, a curved muscle that separates the chest from the abdomen, which massages the nearby organs as it moves, helping with digestive function. Fully engaging that big muscle is called "diaphragmatic breathing" (and sometimes "belly breathing"), and that's what you should be going for.

Breathing *slowly* and breathing *through your nose* rather than your mouth, even, whenever possible, during times of exertion. Going back again to how nature designed us, the nose is built to be our primary breathing portal for reasons that range from its germ-filtering abilities to its power, as the initiator of the inhale, to funnel more oxygen to our cells. Mouth breathing is your backup ventilation system. It's for those times when you're running from a bear or escaping a fire or when you have a cold and your nose is clogged—not for when you're simply sitting in a chair or sleeping. Nose breathing is not only normal, but it also helps you sleep better, get up the stairs without panting, exercise harder and longer, and even have better teeth (we'll tell you why later in this chapter).

Breathing to *maximize CO_2 tolerance.* Inhaling brings in the oxygen that feeds every cell in your body; exhaling expels the waste product of that process, carbon dioxide. Oxygen, good; carbon dioxide, bad. At least that's what most of us have been taught—but it's not entirely true. Yes, we must expel CO_2, but we also depend on it to prompt hemoglobin, the protein in the blood that delivers oxygen to the places it's needed, to release all that O_2. It follows, then, that the more CO_2 you can tolerate (i.e., the longer and slower your exhales), the more oxygen you'll be able to utilize.

The fact that breathing is the second in our lineup of Vital Signs is no accident. Effective breathing is intimately connected to almost all the other nine Vital Signs. As mentioned earlier, it's going to help you sleep better (Vital Sign 10). It will also help you get more out of your walks (Vital Sign 4), inject energy into mobilizations for other Vital Signs, and, if you have pain (neck pain especially—see Vital Sign 5), help you treat it yourself. Although it's true that no one has ever had to teach you to inhale and exhale—you got that skill set all on your own—it's also true that both science and experience tell us that retraining yourself to breathe better can improve your life in a vast number of ways. Research has also shown that people with a healthy lung function live longer. We'll talk more about all that in the pages to come, but first let's check out how well you do with CO_2.

Assessment: Breath-Hold Test

Mostly, you can tell how well you're breathing just by paying attention to something you usually don't ever think about. Are you breathing all the way down into your trunk, or are you breathing up in your chest and neck? Are you drawing air in through your nose or pulling it in through your mouth? The answers should be obvious. Your CO_2 tolerance, though, is not as easy to assess, so we've got a test for you. It's called the Breath-Hold Test or BOLT (Body Oxygen Level Test), and it was popularized by Patrick McKeown, an Irishman who goes around the world training people—elite athletes among them—how to breathe more efficiently.

The test involves holding your breath until you feel an urgent and compelling need to take in more air. It won't provide exact numbers like a lab test, but it will give you a fairly good idea of your ability to endure higher levels of CO_2 and set a benchmark for you to improve upon. If you get a low score, you might want to start looking at other issues in your life to see if breathing might be part of the problem. For instance, people with low BOLT scores tend to be snorers and quickly get out of breath when exercising or even just carrying the laundry up the stairs.

PREPARATION

This test should be taken while you're hanging around doing nothing, not after you've just come in from a walk or climbed a rock wall. That is, your breathing should be regular and not at all elevated. You'll need access to a second hand, on a watch or other timepiece. If using a stopwatch, start it before you begin the test so you don't have to fidget with it and attend to your breathing at the same time. Just note the time you start. Also, take note that, despite the name of the test, what you're actually doing is emptying out your lungs and holding an exhale.

THE TEST

Sitting or standing calmly, inhale normally through your nose. Exhale normally through your nose, then pinch your nostrils shut. Hold your breath until your body starts to get a little twitchy and you feel you must breathe. Note how many seconds from the time you clamped and unclamped your nose.

WHAT YOUR RESULTS MEAN

The number of seconds you held your breath is your score.

Below 10 seconds—Your CO_2 tolerance is way below normal; you'll need to work to catch up.

10–20 seconds—This is a good starting place, but you'll need to grow your ability to deal with discomfort.

20–30 seconds—Getting close to what is considered normal.

30–40 seconds—Everyone should eventually land in this range, considered normal.

Before you get anxious about not being "normal," consider that many factors of daily living can conspire to make us poor breathers. But breathing is something we can all do and, with practice, improvement comes relatively quickly. As we'll note again and again throughout this book, there's no shame in getting a low score. You're just looking at a starting point for gauging your improvement.

WHEN SHOULD YOU RETEST?

Give yourself a week of doing the physical practice, then try the BOLT test again. Test once more after another week. After that, retest as you see fit to check whether you've improved.

A Roadmap to Better Breathing

When we think about breathing, if we think about it at all, we think about how to keep the show running. Breathing = life. But what if breathing didn't just allow you to live, but allowed you to *really* live—as in living life to the fullest? That's what happens when you improve your breathing habits. To understand how we're able to make such a bold claim, it helps to know a little bit about what's going on in that body of yours every time you bring in a lungful of air. Here's a synopsis of what happens.

The impulse to breathe begins in your brain, which sends a message to your diaphragm and other breathing muscles, telling them to contract. The contraction pulls down on the lungs, creating a negative pressure that draws air in (whether it be through your nose or mouth), down your throat and trachea, and into the bronchial tubes, where it eventually spills out into the lobes of your lungs. In the far reaches of the lobes are microscopically thin bubbles called "alveoli." This is where the action starts to happen. Oxygen slips through the alveoli into the adjoining capillaries, where it meets up with red blood cells. The O_2 then hops on the back of the red blood cell protein hemoglobin and, pushed along by the beat of your heart, is charioted away to the cells in your muscles and organs. Once delivered, the oxygen is swept into little factories in the cells (called "mitochondria") and used to create energy. It's that energy, ATP, that drives your every bodily function and move. A by-product of this energy production is carbon dioxide, which ultimately gets swept out of the body as you exhale.

Carbon dioxide, however, is not just the shavings left on the floor of the woodshop. We must get rid of it—too much CO_2 and we won't be able to function—but first it has an important role to play. In 1904, a Danish scientist by the name of Christian Bohr discovered that carbon dioxide turns the blood acidic, which prompts hemoglobin to slough off the oxygen it picked up from the lungs. The upshot is that carbon dioxide isn't just a waste product. It actually makes more oxygen available to the body. Which is why when you really need extra oxygen—say you're walking up a hill or skiing down one—the heat generated by your exertion creates more CO_2, resulting in more oxygen release to fuel your working muscles.

Bohr's discovery led to the practice of increasing CO_2 tolerance. The longer you can hang on to carbon dioxide in your system, the more oxygen you'll be able to utilize, and the more oxygen you're able to utilize, the more energy you'll have available for whatever it is you want to do. Climbing the stairs with groceries, climbing a 2,000-foot rise on your bike. Either one. Because lack of oxygen is usually not the obstacle. Most of us can pull in air fairly efficiently, saturating our blood with O_2. Even when we're just breathing quietly, the tank is full. What we don't always do as efficiently is *access* that oxygen, a problem that holding on to CO_2 longer can help solve. That's why when someone having a panic attack is hyperventilating—rapid breathing that floods the system with oxygen but doesn't seem to satisfy oxygen hunger—they are often handed a paper bag. Breathing into the bag sends carbon dioxide back into the system, recalibrating the CO_2 to O_2 balance.

Breathe for Stability and Energy

If you've ever watched a weightlifting competition where brawny athletes hoist massive hunks of iron overhead, you've probably been struck by how much strength it takes to get those things up in the air. And it does. But it also takes something else: good breathing technique. One of the Olympians we've worked with, Wes Kitts, found that out the hard way. Wes actually passed out while competing in the Pan American Games, only to come back three years later and set an American record for the snatch (raising a barbell up in one continuous motion) at the 2020 Tokyo Olympics. One of the keys to his success was learning to use breath to create stiffness in his trunk while, at the same time, shuttling oxygen to his working muscles.

Granted, Wes isn't your garden-variety guy (his record-setting lift was 390 pounds), but what he was able to do—handle load and ventilate simultaneously—is something everyone should be able to do, whether it's at an Olympic level or when you just want to carry a big load of firewood into the house without feeling faint. That's the definition of a useful human.

There are many things you'll want to do in life that you'll be able to accomplish with greater ease and without messing up your body if you use breath constructively. Your neighbor asks you to help lift his couch. You're moving a box of junk into your garage. You're pulling a bag of golf clubs out of your trunk. You want to be like Wes Kitts (but are starting with 10-pound dumbbells). All those movements are going to go well when you breathe right.

It works like this. When you breathe diaphragmatically, drawing air into the whole of your trunk—expanding your ribs, chest, and belly versus shallowly breathing into your neck and chest—you create a stiffness around the spine that enables your body to handle load or other physical challenge without having to twist or flex or otherwise angle into positions that are at best untenable, at worst injurious. In a sense, mostly everyone intuitively knows that air provides stability since mostly everyone, when faced with exertion, will hold their breath. For instance, anytime we test balance by asking people to raise their arms overhead and stand on one leg, 100 percent of them hold their breath while doing it.

Say we were to hand you a four-year-old child and ask you to hold her out in front of you like a log. The next thing you'll likely do—without even thinking about it—is take a big inhale and hold it to create a big stiff air bag in your trunk that will protect the spine from the demand of holding a weight. That's a good thing. Being able to create what's called "intra-abdominal pressure" when you need to is a natural safety measure. But pretty soon you'll have to breathe again (especially if you begin to move), so you'll go from breath hold to breath hold until finally your brain tells you you can't retain the level of stability in your trunk and get enough oxygen for the task if you're breathing that way. You'll have to put her down. Your brain has just basically short-circuited your ability to generate force. It's not that you're not strong enough to hold the child; it's just that the brain is highly protective of breathing, so it will downregulate force in favor of breathing. If you can breathe, then whether or not you can hold the child will depend on your level of strength. But strength doesn't even come into play if you can't ventilate.

All this being said, there is some value in holding your breath when the time is right. For instance, breath-holding exercises—also known as "hypoxic training"—can increase your CO_2 tolerance. However, when it comes to daily life, the first step to becoming a good breather, not a breath-holder, is to simply be conscious of the fact that you need to keep inhaling and exhaling at all times and that you need to take full, spacious breaths, not pull in wimpy little wisps of air. You'll see that as you practice the breathing techniques in this chapter, you'll develop the habit of both noticing your respiration and doing it better.

LAIRD AND GABBY'S
EXCELLENT BREATHING ADVENTURE

Swimming back and forth underwater carrying a heavy dumbbell in one hand. Repeatedly jumping from the bottom of the pool up to the surface, this time with dumbbells in both hands. Oh, and doing each exercise with only one breath. It's not everyone's cup of tea, to be sure, but these tests of breath holding coupled with movement have made a, um, splash in the fitness world. As part of XPT, a breathe-move-recover workout plan cocreated by the married couple Gabrielle Reece and Laird Hamilton, the pool exercises use the added difficulty of being underwater to challenge your ability to manage very high levels of CO_2.

Laird, a pioneering big-wave surfer and coinventor of tow-in surfing, and Gabby, a former professional volleyball player, now a sportscaster and podcaster, started doing breath workouts in their own home pool before adding it to their challenging XPT protocol. The idea for adding in weights to increase the difficulty of underwater breath training (essential for someone like Laird, who can end up under the churn of a thirty-foot breaker) came to them when one of their daughters, five at the time, popped up to their pool's surface holding a dumbbell. A new workout was born.

To be clear, we know the body has plenty of oxygen available during these types of exercises; it's the rising CO_2 that drives people to the surface. "People think they're out of air and that they need to come up and breathe, but actually they don't; they're okay," says Gabby. "After a while, they start to understand that the only difference between doing one jump or four jumps without a breath is their ability to be efficient and relaxed. It teaches you some harmony with primal discomfort."

The technical term for this kind of workout is "dynamic apnea training"—limiting air while also moving (*apnea* derives from the Greek word meaning "want of breath"). You can test this for yourself on your local sidewalk. Set a short destination—maybe the closest corner—

then prepare to walk by taking a big breath. Hold the breath as you move forward, only stopping and releasing it when you feel you must inhale again. When you feel you can move again, repeat the breath hold-and-release as many times as necessary until you reach your destination. How many breaths did it take? How long did you have to recover before you could hold your breath and walk again? The more effective you become at accessing the available oxygen in your bloodstream, the faster you'll be able to complete the walk. This is the same principle that helps athletes get an edge over the competition, so you can see why this style of breath training has become so popular with the best ones in the world.

And Gabby sees the benefits as stretching way beyond sports performance. "I'm of the belief that if you can put yourself in productive and helpful but uncomfortable situations on a regular basis, it's good for stress management, which extends to family, work, and self-observation," she says. "And what I love about breathing is it's free and you can do it anywhere. It's one of the most powerful tools we have."

Put Yourself in the Best Possible Position

In the training world, we live by the words of physical therapist Gray Cook, who coined this phrase: "If you can't breathe in a position, you don't own that position." But those words of wisdom apply to *all* positions, in the gym, out of the gym. On occasions when you need to be in a somewhat awkward or taxing position—say, putting your luggage in the overhead compartment or flipping your mattress—spacious, diaphragmatic breathing can help keep you safe and give you the energy you need to meet the demands of that position. You also want to be breathing this way when you're *not* under duress—it's just good, healthy respiration.

Good body positioning can't be divorced from good breathing. Whenever possible, try to make decisions about your posture so as to be able to maintain the integrity of your breathing function. Positions that let you breathe more easily and effectively are better, more functional shapes. And, in fact, if you can't inhale into your whole trunk, it's a sign that your body isn't organized properly.

"Organized" is a term we often use to refer to how you arrange your body. For instance, standing with your hips slightly jutted out and your shoulders back is a way of organizing your muscles, bones, and joints. So is sitting with your torso angled forward. How you're organized is your position/posture. What you want to aim for is an organization of body parts that allows you to take a full breath. The breath, in fact, can be a bellwether of the effectiveness of your body's position. Sometimes we don't realize that we're standing or sitting or moving in ways that limit our mechanical efficiency or functional output. To see what we mean, try this:

Sit in a chair with your upper back rounded and shoulders slumped, just like your mother always told you not to. From this slouchy position, let your shoulders roll in slightly toward your chest. Now take a moderately deep breath. Note how it feels. Next, reorganize your body and choose a position where you think you can take a bigger breath. Once again, take a moderately deep inhale. Feel the difference? The first breath probably felt constricted, while the second breath—if you arranged your body into an easy but fully upright position—probably felt like you were giving your whole body a good dose of air.

For years we've been taught that slumping and slouching were mostly a sin of aesthetics, but as it turns out they're more a crime against the pulmonary system. If you can't take a nice full breath in a position, you're not going to be able to efficiently move air in and out of your body. You may be organizing yourself into positions and practicing movement patterns that don't allow you to fully take advantage of your body's incredible physiology. What's more, the restrictive nature of your positioning will likely make you default to breathing into just your neck and chest. That's sort of like breathing through a straw and can potentially be a component of neck and other types of pain, as well as lead to teeth grinding and headaches.

The bottom line is this: Instead of worrying about your posture, simply ask yourself, "Can I breathe well in this position?" If the answer is yes, your body positioning is just fine. You're getting the air you need, using your breathing apparatus as it's intended to be used, and not likely putting undue strain on your body. Win-win-win. Checking your breathing is a strategy you can (and should) apply to many daily situations. While sitting behind a desk working on your computer. During your Peloton workout. When you need to pick up something heavy like a squirming child or recalcitrant pet. The better able you are to effectively breathe and create that pressurized chamber that supports your spine, the more capable you'll become.

Slow Down and Keep Your Mouth Shut

We mean this in the nicest way. There's good evidence that slowing down your breathing and breathing through your nose will net you a host of health benefits, including improving your body mechanics. And once you start thinking about the difference between nose and mouth breathing, you'll start to notice examples of both all around you, in popular culture, in sports, everywhere. If you're a *Star Wars* fan, go back and watch the desert battle between Rey (actor Daisy Ridley) and Kylo Ren (Adam Driver) in *Episode IX: The Rise of Skywalker.* At the start of the scene, Rey is visibly breathing hard through her mouth, but then she closes it, takes a few deep breaths through her nose, pulls out her lightsaber, and executes a breathtaking flip over the fast-approaching, monster-winged flying TIE vehicle. All powered by a few controlled inhales and exhales through her nose.

Okay, that's fiction, but one has to believe that Ridley, as an actor, was on to something. From the annals of real life, look to mixed martial arts fighter Conor McGregor's bout against Floyd Mayweather. During the fight, both of them had their mouths shut, but then McGregor opens his mouth in order to keep up with his breathing and ends up losing the round. Many people have noted that when Eliud Kipchoge became the first person to run a marathon in under two hours, he was breathing through his nose at the finish line. Coincidence? There are many reasons we think not.

First let's talk about why you should care if you are not interested in fighting, running, or any other athletic pursuit (and maybe you even hate *Star Wars*!). It is well established that humans were intended to primarily breathe through their noses. When it comes to filtering out bacteria and infectious bugs, humidifying the body, and warming up air so it slides more easily through the bronchial tubes, nose breathing handily beats mouth breathing. But as James Nestor documents so well in his book *Breath: The New Science of a Lost Art,* evolutionary forces conspired to shrink both our mouths and sinuses, making it harder to breathe through the nose (and crowding our teeth—ancient skulls reveal there was once no need for orthodontia). This is the state of affairs for just about everyone, but some people have complicating factors like allergies or structural differences that turn them into mouth breathers in the real, not the "they're dopey," sense of the word.

Mouth breathing is associated with a number of ills, including insomnia, sleep apnea, snoring, allergies, congestion, gas and bloating (from sipping air while you're also chomping on food), higher blood pressure, and even poor dental health. One study found that mouth breathers had more plaque and the type of bacteria that causes cavities. Breathing through your mouth can also trigger musculoskeletal issues. Mouth breathers tend to jut their heads forward, increasing the weight on the spine. We also see a lot more stiffness in the jaw and in the neck when people inhale through their mouth because, when you mouth breathe, you default to using the musculature in the upper chest and neck to inflate the lungs rather than using the primary ventilation engine of the diaphragm.

This shallow method of breathing can be stressful, too. Short, sharp mouth breaths trip the sympathetic nervous system, the stress-response network that puts the body in fight-or-flight mode. Using the "power assist" breathing muscles of the neck creates a state of arousal that can increase heart rate and blood pressure and just generally take a toll on the body. The fight-or-flight system is meant to work in short-term bursts, but instead you've got your brain thinking it should be using a turbo supercharger to run your body all day long. That's a lot of inefficiency and extra energy expenditure.

Granted, there are times when you're going to have to breathe through your mouth. If you're not used to walking up a hill or running for a bus, you're going to need to mouth breathe to satisfy your oxygen needs. It's nearly impossible to swim without mouth breathing. Some athletes, however, have trained themselves to breathe through their noses even when making extreme demands on their muscles. A Colorado State University study found that runners who practiced working out while nose breathing for six months were able to retain the same aerobic benefits while ultimately being able to preserve energy during their runs. With some training, we've seen some of our athletes be able to work out at heart rates around 90 percent of their max while still breathing through their noses!

Whether you want to work toward this type of goal or not, it's worth your while to learn to nose breathe for everyday living if you don't naturally do so already. Nose breathing almost always triggers more efficient breathing mechanics, including inhaling with the diaphragm as you're meant to. And you don't even need to train for it. You just close your mouth.

The payoff is notable. Nose breathing, for instance, has been shown to reverse almost all the bad effects of mouth breathing, curing sleep apnea and snoring, righting breathing problems caused by congestion and allergies, and improving blood pressure. A few things are happening here. When you inhale through your nose, nitric oxide (NO) is released in the nasal cavity. This gas is a vasodilator, meaning it widens the blood vessels, enabling more—18 percent more—oxygen to flow to your cells. It can also increase your lung capacity, which is no small thing: The bigger and more efficient your lungs, the longer you're likely to live, according to the Framingham Heart Study, a long-running investigation into cardiovascular risk factors that began in 1948.

Another benefit of breathing through your nose is that you're going to be more likely to take the kind of spacious, torso-expanding breaths we talked about earlier. These kinds of breaths reach into the lower depths of the lungs, where they turn on the parasympathetic nervous system. The parasympathetic system is our "rest and digest" control center, preparing the body to do those very things. It is, in other words, calming and allows us to take care of the business of nourishing the body. This is why meditative practices call for deep breathing, and the reason "take a deep breath" is not an empty platitude but a valuable piece of advice. It's not necessarily that you want to live in this parasympathetic blissed-out state all the time. We need to be able to go from state to state, press on the gas pedal and function in high gear when warranted, then hit the brakes as needed. But when you mouth breathe, a lot of your body mechanics stay on the hit-the-gas mode when you're trying to slow down.

If you combine nose breathing with expansive breathing, then add in slower breathing, you'll have hit the trifecta. (It's actually the quadfecta, if you consider that taking bigger breaths can help you avoid neck and shoulder pain—see page 62.) Slower breathing—both slower inhaling and exhaling—develops CO_2 tolerance and increases blood flow to the brain, all the while helping the lungs, as Nestor puts it, "soak up" more oxygen from the air we suck in. It may sound complicated, so many different elements, but as you'll see when you try out the physical practices in this chapter, it all comes together quite easily. And breathing well is habit-forming.

BLOWING PAIN AWAY

While it's happening to you, pain seems like a thing unto itself, a distinct entity, a force. But physical pain is actually your brain's *perception* of what's happening to your body. It's a signal sent down the wire meant to telegraph that something is wrong. How that signal is interpreted or even noticed can vary dramatically. Consider, for instance, Paul Templer's account of feeling no pain in the face of severe injuries, a story that took place on the Zambezi River in Zimbabwe, near Victoria Falls. Templer, a river guide at the time, was leading boats full of tourists through a particular stretch of the Zambezi known for its population of hippos, crocodiles, and cape buffalo, aggressors all. Still, it's the site of regular guided canoe tours and considered relatively safe.

Not that day. A two-ton bull hippo lifted one of the canoes in the air, flinging Templer's colleague into the water. Attempting to help the guy, Templer found himself in the bull's mouth. The hippo proceeded to practically swallow him, shake him like a rag doll, throw him into the air and catch him again, and chomp on Templer with his knifelike tusks. By the time the guide was rescued, he had forty puncture wounds—including one so deep his lung was visible—and a shredded arm that he'd go on to lose on the operating table. And yet, after he had some first aid, Templer set about making sure all the clients were safe and has said he didn't feel the pain (though he certainly did later).

Part of why this story resonates with us is that Juliet, too, was attacked by a hippo in the same place and around the same time (mid-1990s) as Templer. It was 1997 and she and her teammates were celebrating a win at the nearby extreme rafting world championships with a canoe safari on a calmer part of the Zambezi. On day three, they reached a series of channels, and when their guide asked the women (which included Juliet's not entirely adventurous mother) if they wanted to take the "Hippo City" or the "Hippo Bronx" route, the majority voted for the tougher Bronx byway. Moments later a hippo charged Juliet's boat, flipping her and a teammate into the water—a fifty-yard swim from the closest island, with a possibility of crocodiles and more hippos en route and notoriously nasty cape buffalos waiting on the shore. They swam for their lives. Juliet ended up with only a scratch, and all too aware of what could have been, plus a deep empathy for Templer and his plight.

Sorry for the digression (but good stories, no?), and to get back to the original point, Templer's experience, or should we say nonexperience, of what should have by all rights felt excruciating demonstrates that it's possible to interrupt or change how your brain makes sense of what is happening in your body. Something can be wrong, but it doesn't always have to cause us extreme discomfort. We don't know the particulars of how Templer was able to sidestep pain for a time, but we do know that breathing can be used as a desensitization tool—if not when you're staring down a furious hippo, most certainly when you've got something like a nagging backache.

Or are having a baby. One critical component of the Lamaze method, which has been around since the 1950s, is deep breathing to help the impending mothers endure the pain of childbirth. So the notion that breathing modulates the perception of pain isn't new (and most certainly goes back way further than the fifties), though we're just beginning to understand a little bit about how it works. Which brings us to Wim Hof.

No discussion of breathwork would be complete without introducing you to Hof. If you don't already know about "The Iceman," famed throughout the world, here are a few of the Dutchman's accomplishments: climbing both Mt. Kilimanjaro and Everest in shorts, and setting Guinness World Records for, among other things, swimming under ice, running a half-marathon barefoot in Finland, and sitting immersed in a box of ice for close to two hours. Oh, he also ran a marathon in the Namib Desert without drinking any water.

Hof would tell you that his ability to feel no pain in the cold or heat is not superhuman, but rather owing to his ability to harness something quite ordinary: breathing. His Wim Hof Method combines breathwork—cycling through rounds of thirty to forty deep breaths and some breath holds for about six minutes—with cold exposure and mental focus, but it's the breathing that makes the other two possible, especially the cold exposure. "The breathing generates heat through the intercostal muscles, and it also increases your pain tolerance," writes Hof in *The Wim Hof Method*. How exactly it increases tolerance of savage subzero temperatures was something researchers at Wayne State University looked at by studying Hof up close. After suiting Hof up in special apparel that exposed him to both hot and cold, they found that Hof was able to change his biochemistry at will, stimulating the release of brain chemicals that inhibit pain signals in the body. And it isn't just Hof who can do it; some of his followers have participated in studies that found that they, too, could alter their body's biochemistry.

Other research also suggests that breathing can make it easier to bear the pain of extreme temperatures. One study measured how well a group of people were able to tolerate increasing heat under different conditions. Each person had a heating device applied to their forearm while taking slow, deep breaths; breathing normally; breathing rapidly; playing a video game (distraction); or hooked up to a biofeedback machine. The heat was raised incrementally until the person was no longer able to stand it. By the end of the study, it was clear: Pain threshold was significantly higher during the deep, slow breathing and the biofeedback (which also involved slow breathing) protocols. Distraction had a positive effect on pain tolerance, too, but not as significant as breathing.

How does the deep, slow breathing work? While the researchers—scientists at the Université de Sherbrooke in Quebec—couldn't say for sure, they noted that conscious breathing increased activity in the parasympathetic "rest and digest" system, slowing heart rate and otherwise blissing out the body. The ability of breath to keep us in this relaxed state may just be why it helps with pain, especially when you consider the alternative. When the body is in fight-or-flight, high-arousal, twitchi-ness mode, the brain pays attention to subtle input, making it more likely that you'll be aware of pain signals coming in via the central nervous system. The idea that the nervous system, breath, and mental percep-tion are all intertwined is actually an idea that has been around for years. The celebrated yogi master B.K.S. Iyengar once said, "Nerves are king of the breath and the breath is the king of the mind." What we take that to mean is that if you can control your breathing, you can control your mind. And if you can control your mind, you can influence how con-scious you are of pain signals.

Physical Practice: Breathing Exercises and Mobilizations

A large part of becoming a better breather is simply noticing when you're holding your breath or when you're bringing in quick, shallow wisps of air. Now that you know the definition of broke, you can fix it. We also live by the doctrine that practice makes not perfect, but permanent. These exer-cises are just the kind of practice we mean, designed not only to change your habitual style of breathing but also to create physiological change in the body.

In some ways you may already be doing them. You may have noticed that the Vital Sign 1 mobilizations (and all the mobilizations in the book, for that matter) include breathing instructions. Inhaling, exhaling, and holding your breath as you contract and relax your muscles let you hit two birds with one stone. Part of your breathing practice can also be found in the chapter on Vital Sign 4—walking. Combining breathing exercises with your walks shortens your to-do list. And this isn't just about multi-tasking. These things relate to one another. Breathing affects how you move and moving affects how you breathe.

We also have three stand-alone practices for you. One involves solely sitting and breathing; the other two are mobilizations. If you can, work up to practicing them daily.

One last thing before you begin. There are a lot of different breathing practices out there, ranging from yoga pranayama and box breathing (used by the Navy SEALs, it involves inhaling, holding, exhaling, holding) to the Wim Hof Method. If you're interested in going further, we urge you to explore other breathing techniques and add them to the practice we recommend here.

Morning Spin-Up

This is a great way to start your morning. Take the time before the day becomes chaotic to sit quietly and just breathe. We're treating this breath practice like a skill session. You may find that your breathing musculature gets tired after a minute or so. This is normal! It's also okay to feel a little luminous or tingly. Remember: You are just breathing here! If the feeling gets too uncomfortable, take a one-minute break and start back up again. The ideal is to do three to five rounds of this breathing. There is a ton of interesting physiology to play with here. You're using your breathing to improve the range of motion of your ventilation systems. Here's what to do:

Set a timer for two minutes or have a timing device available. While sitting on a chair or, preferably, cross-legged on the floor, or even lying down, take a full breath in through your nose, expanding your chest, ribs, and belly. Treat each breath like it is going to be a record inhale! Relax and exhale fully, saying "huh" as you release the air (don't blow). Don't pause between your exhales and inhales. Repeat for two minutes. Now repeat the practice, only this time exhale fully then hold as long as possible without inhaling. When you feel the need to breathe, inhale and repeat for another two minutes. Alternate these sequences as many times as you desire. Do three to five rounds and you've just worked your way into a meditation practice.

Trunk Mobilization

If you're wound up, hassled, worried about your family, your job, etc., do not stop, do not pass go, just hit this mobilization. What makes it so effective at combating stress is that it stimulates the vagus nerve through both outside physical pressure and the act of breathing. That shifts the body into parasympathetic ("rest and digest") territory and provides a calming effect. Plus, it's a great way to practice the long exhales and boost CO_2 tolerance.

Lie facedown on the floor atop a roller or larger ball (like a volleyball) placed just below your ribs and pressing on your abdomen, arms in front of you. Inhale through your nose for four seconds and hold your breath for four seconds, while contracting your abdominals. Then exhale for five or more seconds as you relax your trunk. Take a big breath or two in between contract and relax cycles. Next, move side to side on the roller/ball as you breathe slowly in and out. If you find an area that's stiff or "off" while on the spot, contract the muscles there as you breathe in for four seconds, then relax for eight seconds as you breathe out. Repeat as many times as needed for a max of about ten minutes.

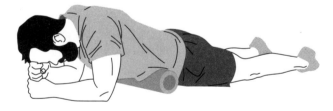

While this exercise can feel strange and intense,
better trunk function awaits in just a few minutes.

T-Spine Mobilization 1

This is another way to practice good breathing while also loosening up the trunk so you can take fuller breaths. "T-spine" is shorthand for thoracic spine, the mid and upper part of your back. Stiffness in the T-spine,

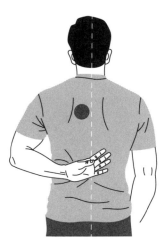

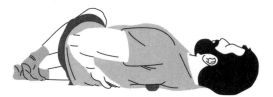

This is a two-for-one: mobilizing the back and working a crucial shoulder shape!

besides inhibiting breathing, puts pressure on the lower spine, potentially causing pain. Creating more movement in the T-spine is a great way to restore a ton of hidden capacity to your body.

Lie on your back and place a small ball behind you on the right side in the middle of your back, somewhere between your spine and your shoulder blade. Begin by just seeing if you can take a full breath in and out in this position. Then, if desired, raise your hips off the ground to increase the pressure on your back. (Remember, only modify to the point where you can still breathe and are not holding your breath.) Now place your right arm under your low to mid back. Gently rock back and forth over the ball taking long slow breaths as you work the ball down the length of your shoulder blade. Repeat on the other side. The pressure from the ball will likely feel more intense in some areas than others. Keep breathing and exploring up to five minutes on each side.

Nose-Breathing Walk
See page 123.

EXTRA CREDIT: TAPE YOUR MOUTH CLOSED

After James Nestor's book *Breath* came out, there was practically a run on athletic tape as people were inspired to use adhesive to ensure they were nose breathing while asleep. Does it work? Reports are that snorers stop snoring, it corrects sleep apnea, and people are getting better, higher-quality sleep. We have heard stories of mouth breathers waking up in the morning with high lactate levels, an indication of stress. Taping is a remedy for this (as is practicing nose breathing while walking—page 123—to help reinforce the habit).

While it sounds drastic, scary even, our own experience with it has been that it feels safe and works well. We followed Nestor's advice, simply using a postage-stamp-size square of fabric tape and taping the mouth horizontally. Put the tape in place before you turn out the lights. If it feels too claustrophobic, go gradually. Try it for ten minutes, then twenty, then work up to sleeping with your mouth taped all night.

THE LUDDITE AND MRS. GADGET

In a world brimming with high-tech fitness gizmos, Kelly has a secret: He's an analog guy. Well, it's not really a secret, since it's as plain as the watch on his wrist—a classic, no bells-and-whistles timepiece. He's a fan of gadgetry and apps but, with a few exceptions, mostly for other people. Juliet, on the other hand, is a believer in the old maxim "What gets measured gets managed," so she's a devotee of both devices and apps that allow you to track fitness and health data and work to improve your stats. At any given time in her life, she's tracking (what seems like) a hundred pieces of data. For her, it's informative and, most of all, fun.

Because of our personal differences on fitness tech, we're agreed on this: There's no right or wrong here. If a smartwatch or an app or any other kind of breathing trainer, data gatherer, or fitness tracker helps you do what you need to do, we are all for it. If you don't feel you need it, don't worry—you're not missing out. It really is an individual choice. If you are interested in checking some out, here are four that we particularly like.

APNEA TRAINER—The word "apnea" refers to temporary cessation of breath. This app guides you in breath-holding exercises that increase CO_2 tolerance.

CORE BY HYPERICE—The Core is a small device you hold in your hand that uses lights and vibrations to guide you in different breathing and meditation exercises. It has biosensors that track your heart rate and pairs with your phone to track your progress.

GARMIN—This company has so many different variations on the smartwatch, including watches geared toward specific sports. You can get these trackers with various features, including a pulse oximeter (which tracks saturation of oxygen in the blood) and a heart rate monitor.

EXTEND YOUR HIPS

ASSESSMENT
Couch Test

PHYSICAL PRACTICE
Hip Mobilizations

W HEN TRAVELING, WE take an uncommon interest in the security line at the airport. As we inch our way toward the TSA agent, we watch people going through the full-body scanner, standing with legs apart, arms above their head. Then we take note of whose hips are locked into flexion. It's a people-watching game that perhaps only two people consumed with movement health could love, but it also confirms what we see in our work day to day: Most people have limited extension in the hips.

Let's walk this back a bit. Flexion, as you might remember, is when an angle between body parts closes. When you sit, your hip is in *flexion* and the angle between your torso and thigh is approximately 90 degrees, relatively closed compared to when you're standing. When you lunge with your leg behind you, the hip of your straight leg is in *extension* and the angle between your torso and thigh is quite open. Hip extension is the yin to the yang of hip flexion.

We can tell that some people in the full-body scanner are in flexion with their thighs and pelvis rolling forward because they have "banana back," which is exactly what it sounds like. The body curves into an unhealthy banana shape with the torso jutting forward and the back arched, a position that puts strain on the system and makes it difficult to breathe properly.

It's not that people exhibiting banana back in the scanner are in such deep flexion that it's like they're sitting, but even this slight flexion in the hips prevents healthy body alignment. What it also means is that they can't access the hip extension they need to stabilize the body when their arms are overhead. With more extension, they would be able to right the ship, stand straight, and avoid imbalance—and, possibly, pain.

When you think about what humans are built for, it's to get up and down, to walk around carrying stuff, and to swing and throw objects. All these things require hip extension, which gives you a power-push forward. When your hip extension is restricted, it basically truncates the forceful movements that enable you to walk and run with ease and speed, stand up from a squat, and throw a tennis ball far enough to give your dog some real exercise. It's an essential ingredient in good functional movement and, when adequate, also a deterrent against pain. It's what helps you go up and down the stairs and sit through a movie without throbbing knees. It's what enables you to get through being on your feet cooking all day for Thanksgiving or standing all night at a concert without feeling spasms in your back.

We often get asked some variation of the questions, "Say someone is only going to do one mobilization. What should it be? What gives you the most bang for your buck?" What they're essentially asking is, "What's the most important body part?" You might as well ask your aunt, "Which of your three children is your favorite?" Or ask yourself this: "You have two kidneys. Which one are you going to take care of?" Or, because we never get tired of car metaphors, "Are you going to rotate your tires but not check your oil?" It's impractical, right? So let us preface this by saying that we don't believe in just doing one mobilization or singling out one area of the body for care at the exclusion of other parts. However, we will concede that a hip extension mobilization (and preferably several hip extension mobilizations) may have the biggest impact on your everyday functionality. If you had to choose one, this would be it.

Assessment: Couch Test

The best way to determine how well you can extend your hips is to take something called the Couch Test. Before you get excited about a test with "couch" in the title, let us explain that it has nothing to do with lounging around on the sofa (though who wouldn't love that?). Rather, the Couch Test is so named because it's based on a mobilization that involves tucking your knee into the seat of a couch with your shin resting on the couch's back. This mobilization, created by Kelly and popularized when Tim Ferriss included it in his book *The Four-Hour Body*, is easy to work into your life—you can hang out in it while you watch the news or stream a show. The test, though, is actually best performed on the floor (with your shin resting on a wall), with the stipulation that, if it's too difficult, you can also perform the test on the couch.

What the Couch Test measures is both your ability to extend your hips behind you and the range of motion in your quadriceps. When these two movements are normalized, your legs can do everything they need to do. If you've never done lunges or any of the moves in yoga like the Warrior I and II poses, extending your hip in the Couch Test may feel both totally unfamiliar and difficult. Worry not. The restrictions that may prevent you from passing the test with flying colors—restrictions you might not have known even existed—can be alleviated with practice. As with so many of the Vital Signs in this book, we want to bring your awareness to the issue so that you not only work to maintain hip flexibility, but also add hip *in*flexibility to your list of things to check when something goes wrong. Lower back hurts? Knees ache? Your running or walking slows down?

You're bent over while walking? Lack of hip extension could be the reason or a contributing factor.

An important, if perhaps unexpected, aspect of this test is that it calls for you to squeeze your butt as firmly as possible as you extend your hip. What you're doing here is activating your glutes, the large muscles in your butt, and the reason this matters is because extending your hip without control leads to just the kind of banana back you're trying to avoid. Yes, you want to be able to get your leg behind you, but for the move to be both safe and powerful, the hip must work in concert with the glutes. (For more about the glutes, see The Rear View, page 86.) This test doesn't actually take the leg back far into extension; instead, it tests how well you can both extend *and* activate the glutes at the same time. That's how you restore basic movement safely and soundly.

Breathing as you go is also going to contribute to the quality and safety of the position. And what we mean by breathing is taking full breaths through your nose and filling up your trunk with air. If you're in one of the more advanced positions and can't breathe fully, back off and drop back to a simpler move. If you're in the simplest move but can't take that trunk-filling breath, consider this as something to work toward and don't move up until you master it.

PREPARATION

You'll need a clear wall and adjacent floor space and, possibly, a couch. If desired, when doing the test on the floor, use a mat or pillow to cushion the knee of the working leg. Remove your shoes before you begin (or risk scuff marks on the wall).

THE TEST

Because doing this test on the floor and wall is a truer assessment of your hip range of motion than doing it on a couch, start with the floor/wall. If that proves too difficult or you have physical limitations that preclude using the floor, follow the instructions for the couch.

On the floor/wall

Position 1: Place your left knee at the intersection of the floor and the wall and rest your shin on the wall, toe pointed. Place your right knee on the ground in front of you and hold yourself up with your hands on the floor. Your torso should be angled over the floor. Keeping your left knee at the floor/wall intersection, squeeze your butt as firmly as possible and inhale to a slow count of five, then relax your butt as you exhale to a slow count of five. Repeat five times. Switch sides. If this is easy and you are able to squeeze your butt firmly—being able to activate the glutes is an important part of the test—move to position 2. If you don't have a sense of whether you've been able to successfully squeeze your butt, reach around and touch it to make sure it's firm. On the flipside, make sure you can breathe! Ideally, flexing your glutes and taking a breath aren't mutually exclusive.

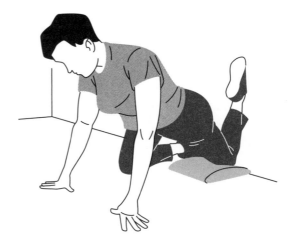

Start with position 1; if you can do it move on to position 2.

Position 2: From position 1, raise your right knee, bend it at a 90-degree angle, and place the foot on the ground in front of you. With your torso angled over the floor and keeping your left knee at the floor/wall intersection, squeeze your butt as firmly as possible and inhale to a slow count of five, then relax your butt as you exhale to a slow count of five.

Repeat five times. Switch sides. If this is easy and you are able to squeeze your butt, move to position 3.

We probably spend most of our time in and around position 2.

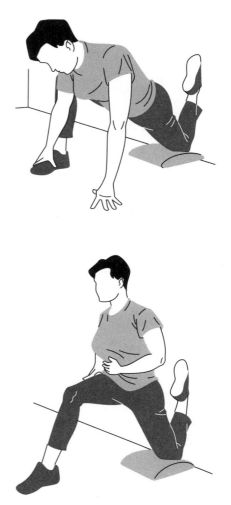

Position 3: From position 2, raise your torso upright so it's as close to parallel to the wall as possible while you keep your left knee at the floor/wall intersection. Squeeze your butt as firmly as possible and inhale to a slow count of five, then relax your butt as you exhale to a slow count of five. Repeat five times. Switch sides.

Moving the torso to more of an upright position really starts to highlight how stiff many of us have become.

On the couch

Position 1: Stand in front of a couch with your back to the seat. Raise your right leg behind you, bend the knee, and tuck it into the seat of the couch near where the back and cushions meet. Rest your shin on the back of the couch, toes pointed. With your torso upright, keep your left foot on the floor and bend your left knee. Keeping your right knee on the seat of the couch, shin against the back of the couch, squeeze your butt

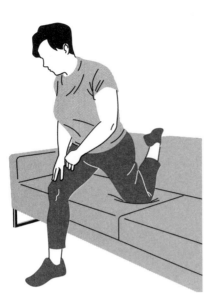

and inhale to a slow count of five, then relax your butt as you exhale to a slow count of five. Repeat five times. Switch sides. If this is easy and you are able to squeeze your butt—being able to activate the glutes is an important part of the test—move to position 2. You can always move your knee away from the back of the couch to make the position more comfortable.

This is the Couch Test as it was originally conceived—you can do it while watching TV!

Position 2: From position 1, bring your left foot onto the couch seat, knee bent at a 45-degree angle. Keeping your right knee on the seat, shin against the back of the couch, squeeze your butt and inhale to a slow count of five, then relax your butt as you exhale to a slow count of five. Repeat five times. Switch sides.

Placing the front foot onto the couch makes the movement more intense.

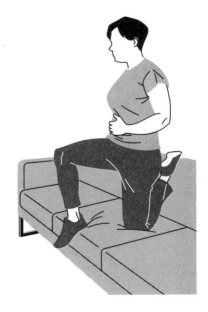

WHAT YOUR RESULTS MEAN

It's very natural to have one hip that's stiffer than the other. Maybe you're left-footed, you drive with your right foot, you push off on your skateboard with the same foot all the time, or you have an old injury that makes one side stiffer than the other. Whatever the reason, it wouldn't be unusual if you were able to get into one position with one leg but not with the other.

On the floor, you hit position 1: You have a fairly good range of motion here, but remember this: As they like to say in physical therapy school, muscles are like obedient dogs. If you're dedicated to their training, they will change. So keep going until you can capably do position 2.

On the floor, you hit position 2: If you can get this much hip extension, consider yourself fairly close to your end range. Keep practicing and soon you'll be able to hit position 3.

On the floor, you hit position 3: Congratulations. You have the kind of hip agility that allows people to excel at sports like running and swimming and offers protection from back and knee pain. Practice will help ensure that you don't lose this essential element of movement.

On the couch, you hit position 1: This is a start. You want to work up at least to baseline.

On the couch, you hit position 2: This is baseline. Even at this point you probably have only a small ability to extend your hip. It could be because you sit a lot of hours and don't walk much. It could also be that you're naturally tight in the area. Give it a try on the floor and see how you do.

WHEN SHOULD YOU RETEST?

You'll naturally retest as you do the Couch Stretch (see page 94). Simply take note of how you progress.

Getting Hip to Extension

Everyone who went through first grade knows that the knee bone's connected to the thigh bone, the thigh bone's connected to the hip bone, and the hip bone's connected to the backbone. Yet even if the words to "Dem Bones" are etched in our memory, most people forget about those connections when it comes to figuring out why their body isn't able to move as well as it's supposed to or why they have discomfort. Just like the song says, everything is connected, and it's because of those connections that the hip, in particular, plays a big role in the body's overall well-being. It even influences how well your big toe performs.

We'll get to that, but let's start by talking about why an inability to extend your hip back into a normal range affects the body part that so many people struggle with: the lower back. The hip has a lot of sway over the back's position even when you're just standing around, and especially when you want to walk fast or run. To get an idea of what happens when the hip can't extend well, try this: Bend over at the waist so your back is at about a 45-degree angle, place your hands in your pockets, and, through the fabric, grab the skin at the top of your upper thigh. (If you don't have pockets, just grab your skin through your clothes.) Now try to stand up straight. You'll find it's difficult to do and that, as your body tries to work around the restriction, you end up either bent over—the problem many older people lacking hip extension have and which increases their risk of falling—or with a hyperextended banana back.

The move, of course, is an exaggeration of what it's like to be lacking in hip extension, but it gives you some idea of why that state of affairs can trigger a cascade of problems. There are two large muscles, the psoas and iliacus, that go from the pelvis to the femur (thigh bone). If they're stiff or shortened, as they tend to be when hip extension is in short supply, they tug on the spine, creating flexion and, if you're standing, banana back. It's a lot of work to keep your back in a swayed, less functional banana back position, potentially leading to lower back fatigue and pain when you move. What's more, when the back must compensate for lack of hip extension, it drags the pelvis forward, making it hard for the diaphragm, pelvic floor, and abdominal muscles to work as effectively as they could. One consequence of that is you're not going to be able to get the ample breaths we talked about in the Vital Sign 2 chapter.

That's what we often see happening in the connected body parts above the hip; there can also be repercussions on the down chain as well. Everyone has some ability to extend their hips, mostly apparent when walking. It doesn't take much extension to stride from your car into work or to saunter down the hall in your house. You step, your leg goes back, and you move forward. Yet if your range of motion is narrow and you're unable to get your leg back very far, the body often turns to alternative ways to find balance and stability, mainly by spinning the leg, knee, and foot outward as you extend your hip backward. Suddenly, you're walking like a duck and complications may ensue. The knee can get stiff and sore, and the ankle—this evolutionary gift that gives our body lift as we move—doesn't track like an ankle should, which can lead to pain as well. If you're a runner, you may end up being a heel striker, someone whose foot's first point of contact is the heel. That isn't necessarily bad; some heel-striking runners do fine, but for others it increases the risk of injury.

Then there's the big toe. The big toe has a big job in the body. One of the things that distinguishes us humans from our primate cousins is our ability to walk upright, and we owe a lot of that to the big toe, which flexes, stiffens, and, as we push off, propels us forward. (If you look at a chimpanzee's foot, you can see that the toes don't align the way human toes do, but chimps are a lot better at using their big toes for grabbing than we are.) But when there's a deficit of hip extension and the foot turns out to compensate, the toe push off is negligible. Conversely, if you have good extension, you can get a lot of power from the toe (runners, power walkers, and hikers take note)—just another reason why being able to nimbly move your leg back is important.

THE REAR VIEW

Because your glutes—the big muscles in your rear—play an important role in hip extension, now is a good time to talk about your butt. One of the jobs of the glutes, which are the largest muscles in the body, is to control the pelvis so that it doesn't pitch forward and cause you to have a swayed banana back—and the strain and instability that come with it. For this reason, it's important to be able to activate—squeeze— the butt when needed, such as when you're doing the Couch Stretch (page 94) or a plank, but also just when you're doing something simple like holding a box or standing for long periods of time. You don't have to keep your butt firm the whole time you're engaged in a daily activity, like using a stand-up desk, for instance. However, checking in with a butt squeeze once in a while is a good way to reset and to make sure you're in a favorable position. So after an hour or two of being on your feet at your desk or a long wait in line at the deli, squeezing your butt will help you check that you're not allowing your pelvis to pitch forward and tug on your spine.

Research shows that glute weakness is associated with knee injuries, chronic lower back pain, shin pain, falls among the elderly, and more. Glute strength, on the other hand, has been shown to remedy many of these same situations. You can really see the effect of how much stability the glutes provide if you experiment with the plank pose, the position at the top of a push-up. If you're in plank and not squeezing your butt, your back would most likely sink, and someone could push on your hips and you'd collapse. But if you're squeezing your butt in the position, suddenly you're like, well, a plank. That same person could sit on you, and you'd stay steady.

If that's not enough to convince you that your back end needs attention, perhaps you care about the shape of your butt—and the number of people getting butt implants these days (the very fact that there is such a thing as butt implants!) says that a shapely ass is indeed a coveted commodity. It just so happens that it's actually very easy to strengthen the glutes and get that nice rounded backside: All you have to do is squeeze. That's what sixteen subjects did in a Wichita State University study published in 2019. The butt-strength guinea pigs simply did butt squeezes for fifteen minutes a day—and it didn't matter if the minutes were broken up, as long as it added up to fifteen. One group did them while seated, five-second squeezes with a brief relaxation in between (essentially isometrics). Another group in the study did an exercise called "bilateral bridges," which involved lying on the floor faceup, knees bent, and raising the hips up, squeezing briefly, then lowering down again. They had the same fifteen-minute protocol.

At the end of the eight-week study, both groups had equal improvements in both hip extension and glute strength, though only the seated glute squeezers showed any increase in the size of their butts. Here's what we love about this study: It shows that you don't have to go to the gym and work out to improve your glute strength and hip extension. While the study subjects did the isometrics sitting down, they'd be just as effective standing up—which means you can do them while waiting in line for coffee, as you wash the dishes, as you brush your teeth. It's really that simple.

INVEST IN YOUR FUTURE (BODY)

In business, we hear a lot about prepping for the future: three-year plans, five-year plans, vision boards to help you imagine the success of your company. In life, we hear a lot about IRAs and 401(k)s and all the ways to save for the "golden years." You know what we never hear a lot about? Anyone's plans to develop the physical skills and capabilities that will allow them to do the things they want to do when they're seventy-five, eighty, ninety, and beyond. Where is the twenty-five-year plan with the end goal of "Hey, I want to be able to walk around Disneyland with my grandkids for two days and not have to rely on anyone else to hoist my luggage into the overhead bin on a plane. I want to still be able to ride my mountain bike and have the strength to get up off the floor if I fall, and shower standing up when I'm ninety-nine"?

One of the things we do with our athletes is look at the event they want to train for, then work backward. We get into the granular details of what the event will entail so that we can help them prepare properly. This is what we should all be doing as we grow older—a deep dive into what old age really looks like and training for it rather than just crossing our fingers and hoping that our genetics are good. You may not be able to prevent a catastrophe like cancer or Parkinson's disease, but there are things you can do to prepare for the years ahead, even if old age is *very* far ahead.

We think that Peter Attia has the right idea. Attia is a physician who created something called the Centenarian Olympics, his answer to the question "Why aren't we training to be kick-ass ninety-year-olds?" Attia came up with the idea after a funeral for a friend's father where mourners lamented that, for ten years before he died, the departed man hadn't been able to engage in the two things he really loved: golf and gardening. The Centenarian Olympics isn't an actual communal sporting event, but rather functions as a personal holy grail. Think about how you want to live your life, take into consideration that the body naturally gets stiffer and weaker with age, and undertake strategies to counter those potential erosions before they set in. If, for instance, you want to be able to play tennis until you drop dead, focus on the strength, balance, and mobility moves that will allow it to happen.

Everything in this book is geared toward seeing you stay active and well into old age. If you add regular exercise into the mix, you're going to fare even better (see page 279 for our take on working out). But the main thing we want to stress is that to be able to keep moving when you're older, you need to get or keep moving now. We can think of no greater example of how nicely that can play out than a trip we took to the Grand Canyon with Juliet's dad, Warren.

It was a physically rigorous trip, sixteen days of paddling the Colorado River, hiking, and sleeping out in the elements. There was a group of us, mostly in our early to late forties at the time; at seventy-six, Juliet's dad was by far the oldest. And yet he did everything we did, though this was no walk in the Grand Canyon National Park. There were sandstorms (we woke up on more than one morning with sand in every orifice) and monsoon rains and days that were 105 degrees and dry. Each morning we loaded up our rafts with dry bags and camping equipment, and we unloaded them every night. During the day we'd run Class IV and V rapids—which means you can't just sit idly by in the boat; you have to paddle. During breaks from the river, we'd take hikes as long as six miles, gnarly hikes that involved climbing and scrambling over rocks.

Warren might have been a little more tired than the rest of us at the end of the day, but he didn't miss out on a thing. When the trip was over, every single one of our fellow travelers was marveling at his agility and stamina. Some of them said that there was no way that their own parents, the same age as Juliet's dad, could have managed the Grand Canyon trip. When asked why he thought he was able to handle the exertion, Juliet's dad said, "Well, I'm sure there's some genetics at work"—not surprising coming from a scientist—"but I've also been moving my entire life."

Naturally, we think it's the latter that made the biggest difference; DNA can only get you so far. The thing is, Warren really invested in his future. He started going to the gym in the 1970s and lifting weights long before either activity was in the national consciousness. He would hike and backpack. He was an early adopter of healthy habits and it's had a big payoff.

So here's how to invest in your own future: Think about all the things you want to do when you're in your senior years. Use your imagination. What will bring you happiness? Write it down to show you're serious about it and to have something to refer back to when your motivation wanes. Then, using this book as your jumping-off point, do what you need to do to retain the physical prowess that will make those things a reality. Start now—before it's too late!

Putting More Glide in Your Stride

If we're designed to have ample extension in the hips, built to extend the hip beyond the midline of our bodies, where did that extension go? As with so many modern ills, hours spent sitting is a major part of the problem. While extension by definition is a lengthening of the tissues that allow the hip to swing back, flexion—the position your hip is in when you sit—shortens and/or stiffens the tissues in the front of the hip and leg. As the body adapts to this formation it's molded into again and again, restriction in the hip is inevitable. And it's not just parking yourself on the couch in front of the TV or working behind a desk all day that perpetuates the tissue shortening. Popular workouts like Peloton and SoulCycle and other activities that put you on a bike or in a boat with a paddle or on a stationary rower for lengthy amounts of time play into what has now become your body's preferred posture.

The great thing about the human body is that it adapts, then it adapts again. You can, in other words, rewild your hip, but it takes a conscious effort. When we look at people in high-level sports environments who are having problems like knee or back pain, one of the things we do is survey the shapes and positions they're moving in throughout the day—and the shapes and positions they're *not* moving in throughout the day. What we almost always see is a dearth of hip extension activities. So it's not just the sitting and the cycling and whatever puts people in flexion; it's the lack of extension. Most of us, even elite athletes, don't have occasion to get our knees behind our hips at a meaningful distance. Unless you do yoga or some other workout that calls for lots of lunging, you probably don't spend any time in this position. Even if you watch someone on an elliptical trainer, which would seem to take the body through a healthy range of motion, you can see that they don't really have to extend their hip while working out on the machine.

When we drill down into the area's anatomy a bit, we can see various repercussions of not practicing hip extension or of lots of sitting (or both). One thing that can happen is that the hip capsule—a bag of connective tissue that attaches the head of the femur (the ball) to the hip socket—can be stiff, a function of it having adapted to the positions it's most often in. Down below, a shortening of the rectus femoris, one of the quadriceps muscles, which crosses the hip joint (it's like the crossbody bag of the upper leg), might be the culprit. There's also a possibility that trouble could lie in the long piece of connective tissue that runs from the top of your foot up over your knee up to your belly. It, too, can become adaptably stiff or short. We don't discount the brain, either. It can be because of an injury or because of practice, but for whatever reason, the brain doesn't allow the body to access a position that you're actually physically capable of getting into. It has a blind spot—though a blind spot that can be removed with the right kind of input.

Bodies often change and we're not always sure why. And, frankly, we don't care why. What we care about is the fastest way to return someone to their native movements, and the good news is that you can make substantial change quickly. Here's an example.

A friend and colleague of ours, strength and conditioning coach Joe DeFranco, was looking for a way to help an NFL running back get his mojo back after knee surgery. Joe worked a hip mobility drill (much like the one that's in store for you later in this chapter) into the athlete's warmup, then had him run a 10-yard sprint. The guy beat his personal record by .05 seconds, his stride opening up immediately after practicing the hip mobility drill. This might seem like a tiny little improvement, but not if you multiply it by 10 (he'd lower his personal best by a half second in the 100) or consider that his job as a running back is to accelerate those first 10 yards on the field.

If you, like probably .000000001 percent of the population (just a guess here), are interested in lowering your running time, this is great news. But what if you're not a runner—why should you care? Because the running back's experience shows that you can make a quick change in how your body moves in the world, whatever that type of movement may be. The episode made a big impact on Joe. "After seeing an elite athlete shave half a second off his 10-yard sprint, it made me think just how important and powerful it is to fully extend the hip. If an elite athlete's body experienced such major change so quickly, what would training end-range hip extension do for the 'Average Joe'?" says Joe. "It was literally that day that hip extension became a primary focus in all my programming for nonathlete clients, and it has had a major impact on 'cleaning up' common issues and complaints. My clients now have better pelvic alignment and less low back, hip, and knee pain."

This isn't an anomaly. Travis Mash is a world-class coach who instituted hip extension mobilizations in his weightlifting athletes' training. When he and Kelly appeared on a podcast together, he gave us some news. "Kelly," he said, "I haven't told you this yet, but you basically cured the back problems at our gym. We started focusing on improving hip extension in our Olympic lifters, and most of the back pain went away." That's what we like to hear!

If we haven't already convinced you that having a fully functional hip is important, let us drive it home with a final pitch. You may walk fine, run regularly without incident, and don't have discernible banana back or other signs that your body is off-kilter. But when you want to scale up— hike a mountain, obtain a personal best in a 5K, kick harder in the pool to leave your lane mate in your wake, walk the hill towns of Tuscany while on vacation—good hip extension is going to be your best friend. It's like taking off a pair of too-tight jeans. You can move, really move.

Even if you have no intention of scaling up in any way, shape, or form, getting your hips into extension is just good basic body maintenance and a way to offset the aging process. You're simply going to be able to move with greater ease. And this is a further reminder that, if you have aches and pains, hip extension is a good place to begin your investigation. We know from our own experience and the experience of others that hip extension mobilizations can remedy seemingly intractable situations.

WHY DO WE HAVE BRAINS? TO MOVE

It's possible that we have brains so that we can contemplate issues like, Why do we have brains? And, of course, it's our wily brains that have helped us—except for the odd angry hippo (see page 67)—dominate the animal kingdom. But some people believe, and we are among them, that the brain's most important job is to direct the body's movements. Columbia University neuroscientist Daniel Wolpert subscribes to that theory, too, and he made the case for it during a TED Talk way back in 2011. As he spoke, Wolpert flashed a photo of sea squirts on the screen, hardly what you'd expect to see in a lecture titled "The Real Reason for Brains." The sea squirt is an exceedingly humble animal, and the particular variety up on Wolpert's screen—opaque with a ribbed, cellulose-like body—looked like an empty water bottle.

Still, rudimentary construction and all, the sea squirt, like us, has a brain and nervous system—at least in the beginning. When young, the animal swims freely around the ocean, but eventually it finds a suitable rock, attaches itself, and stays there for the rest of its life. Once ensconced, the sea squirt ingests its brain and nervous system. Strange, yes, but also quite efficient: Now that it's completely sedentary, the sea squirt doesn't need them anymore. "Movement," Wolpert told his TED Talk audience, "is the most important function of the brain."

Physical Practice: Hip Mobilizations

Most of us use our bodies in asymmetrical ways. It's unlikely that you will spend as much time in hip extension as you do in hip flexion, and no one—least of all us—expects you to. And you don't need to. But sitting less (see Vital Sign 9) and getting your hip into extension daily through some targeted moves will go a long way toward restoring its normal range of motion. There's no magic to it; it's just the simple process of using it so you don't lose it.

The physical practice for greater hip extension involves actually putting your hips into extension (no surprise there), as well as doing some moves to work the stiffness out of the surrounding tissues. Practice them as often as possible. There's also a couple of extra-credit mobilizations we urge you to work into your routine, too. They're not mandatory but are well worth your while.

Couch Stretch
The Couch Stretch is essentially the Couch Test. The only difference is that you do it for longer. Once again, while you'll get the most out of it if you do it on the floor, it's totally acceptable to do it on the couch while you're just hanging out watching your favorite National Geographic spe-

cial (or anything else, of course). We just want you to get your hip into extension; we are open-minded about where you do it.

A few things to remember: Your hips' ability to extend may not be the same on each side. Modify as needed. And don't skip the breathing. As you take a full breath in, you challenge the fascia and connective tissue differently than if you were breathing shallowly or holding your breath. Breathing lets you explore greater ranges of motion. Remember: If you can't breathe in a position, you don't own that position.

Tips for modifying the position: If you find the Couch Stretch difficult to hold for three minutes on each side, do a minute at a time, then go back to it. Or move your knee away from the wall or back of the couch. That will lessen the intensity. Another way to ease up, when you're on the floor in position 1 or 2, is to set a chair in front of you and place your hands on the seat to support your upper body.

On the floor/wall

Position 1 (page 80): Once you're in position: Keeping your right knee at the floor/wall intersection, squeeze your butt and inhale to a slow count of five, then relax your butt as you exhale to a slow count of five. Repeat for three minutes. Switch sides. If this is easy and you are able to squeeze your butt, move to position 2.

Position 2 (page 80): Once you're in position: With your torso angled over the floor and keeping your right knee at the floor/wall intersection, squeeze your butt and inhale to a slow count of five, then relax your butt as you exhale to a slow count of five. Repeat for three minutes, taking breaks as needed. Switch sides. If this is easy and you are able to squeeze your butt, move to position 3.

Position 3 (page 81): From position 2, raise your torso upright so it's as close to parallel to the wall as possible while you keep your right knee at the floor/wall intersection. Squeeze your butt and inhale to a slow count of five, then relax your butt as you exhale to a slow count of five. Repeat for three minutes. Switch sides.

On the couch

Position 1 (page 81): Once you're in position: Keeping your right knee pressed into the seat of the couch and your right shin against its back, squeeze your butt and inhale to a slow count of five, then relax your butt as you exhale to a slow count of five. Repeat for three minutes. Switch sides. If this is easy and you are able to squeeze your butt, move to position 2.

Position 2 (page 82): Once you're in position: Keeping your right knee pressed into the seat of the couch and your right shin against its back, squeeze your butt and inhale to a slow count of five, then relax your butt as you exhale to a slow count of five. Repeat for three minutes. Switch sides.

Quad-Thigh Mobilization

Your quads are one of the largest muscle groups, and they're responsible for a lot of the work your body performs as well as helping to support your weight and move you along throughout your day. Most times, they've also gotten pretty good at staying at the length required for sitting. This mobilization helps restore suppleness to the stiff tissue in the quads. You'll need a foam roller for this mobilization, but a tube-like device (wine bottle, rolling pin, a couple of baseballs taped together) can get you started.

Lie on your stomach with a roller positioned under the top of your right thigh (but really, any real estate from the top of the hip to the knee). Roll slightly to the outside of your right leg; then, keeping your movements slow, roll toward the inside of the leg. Make sure you are working at a pressure that feels significant but still allows you to take a full breath. If the pressure you are using is taking your breath away or you are holding your breath, lighten up on the pressure. Systematically work your way up or down your thigh working from side to side. This may be slightly uncomfortable, which is typical and okay. The rolling should just feel like pleasant pressure. Switch sides. Start with two to three minutes per side, working up to four to five minutes.

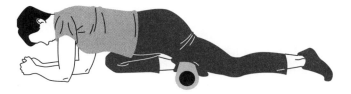

Mobilizing the thigh is probably lowest on the list of fun ways to care for your body. It should be at the top, however.

EXTRA CREDIT: HIP EXTENSION ISOMETRICS

If you can spare a few extra minutes in your day, these are easy to do and very effective. They're isometric exercises—exercises that require contracting and releasing muscles as you go. (If you can make a tight fist, you're making an isometric contraction.) These moves don't work a particular muscle like, say, a biceps curl does. What they do instead is place your body in natural positions, positions that are exaggerated versions of ones you would use in your everyday life. By getting into these positions, and through contracting and releasing while you're in them, you're telling your brain, "Here I am in this position and I'm safe and it's okay and you should allow me to move my body into this position whenever I need to."

Kneeling Isometric

Kneel on the floor with your right leg at a 90-degree angle and your left knee on the floor behind your butt, torso upright, hands on your right knee. Squeeze the

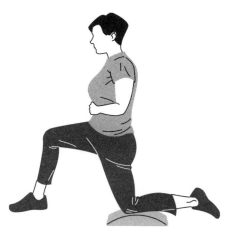

This shape is easy to work into your daily routine. Reminding your brain what your glutes do for a living is a great bonus!

right side of your butt and move your right knee forward as far as you can—it won't go very far with your butt squeezed—and hold the position. Keep your butt tight as you breathe—five slow inhales in, five slow exhales out—for one minute. Make sure you're able to keep the working side of your butt engaged for the entire minute. Switch sides.

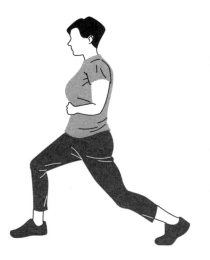

Standing Isometric

Separate your feet with your right foot forward and your left foot back. Bend your right knee slightly and come into a moderate lunge. You should feel tension in the front of your left thigh. Squeeze your butt (on the left side) and hold the position, keeping your butt tight as you breathe—five slow inhales in, five slow exhales out—for thirty seconds. Switch sides.

Since it's practiced while standing, you can do this move anywhere: while waiting for a bus, on the sidelines of a soccer game, and so on.

Couch Isometric (Rear Foot Elevated Mini Lunge)

Stand with your back to the arm of a couch. Step forward with your right foot and rest your left shin on the arm. Bend your right knee into a moderate lunge, squeeze your butt, and hold the position, keeping your butt tight as you breathe—five slow inhales in, five slow exhales out—for thirty seconds. Switch sides.

When performed with movement and weights, this exercise is a staple in training environments across the globe. It's often called the Bulgarian Split Squat.

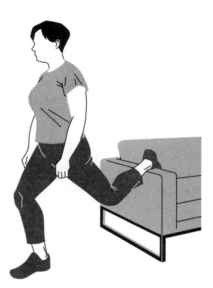

WALK THIS WAY

ASSESSMENT
Steps-Per-Day Inventory

PHYSICAL PRACTICE
Intentional Walks and More-Steps Strategies

> *sedentary* • *adjective*
> *['se-d°n-,ter-ē]*
> *Of inactive habits; pertaining to a sitting posture.*

I F YOU DON'T move much throughout the day, you probably already have a rough idea that you may meet the definition of "sedentary." That's likely why you're here, reading through these pages (or at least we hope so!). But if you're a regular, even an avid, exerciser, you might be surprised to find out that you may qualify as sedentary, too. Many people who are hitting the recommended three-to-five-times-weekly workouts, and even athletes who pile up the training hours, are shocked to learn we consider them basically inert. You might do your stair-climbing workout or CrossFit or Pilates and think, "Sweet! I'm crushing it." But you may then go sit at your legal or computer programming job from 8 a.m.

to 8 p.m., transition to dinner, and cap it off with a session of Netflix. As we've said before, while it's all well and good to knock it out of the park for thirty to sixty minutes a day, if you spend the rest of your waking hours toggling between a chair and sofa, you're in some ways canceling out all the good your workouts are doing.

This is not to put anybody in a corner with a dunce cap and a "sedentary" sign hung around their neck. We get it. When it comes to activity prescriptions—how much, what kind—these are confusing times. Plus, well, life is busy and complicated, and our whole environment is set up to make us sedentary. Desk jobs prevail, technology is alluring, and sometimes movement just doesn't happen. Our goal is to clarify what it really means to be sedentary versus active and, most important, to show you how to *make* movement happen. As you may have guessed by now, it has to do with walking. As a society, we can all stand to move more—we're built to move. Walking is not only an efficient way to get it done, it's also intrinsically tied to the robustness of all the systems and structures in your body. The simple act of walking surpasses any fitness gadget or club membership you can buy; it's the best movement tool available. That said, if physical limitations prevent you from walking, don't give up on the idea of moving more. When we owned a CrossFit gym in San Francisco, we had an adaptive athletics program that enabled people with varying disabilities to find a number of different ways to move, so we know firsthand that there are alternatives to walking out there. All movement is good movement, a ticket out of sedentary living and its potential detriments.

Just exactly what those detriments are has been a subject of some debate. Is sitting really the new smoking? That's a bit of an exaggeration—if you're a human being, you're going to sit at some point; it's inevitable and it's okay. However, the number of hours that the average person sits is unreasonable in terms of our physiology and, research shows, our well-being. In 2010, American Cancer Society researchers published a study based on epidemiological data from 123,216 men and women. What they found was that sitting for a substantial percentage of one's waking day raised the risk of dying *exponentially.* According to the study's metrics, women and men who sit more than six hours a day are 37 percent and 18 percent, respectively, more likely to die before people who sit less than three hours a day. What's more, the negative effects were just as strong in people who exercised regularly. Subsequent studies have had similar results.

"Sitting" has become synonymous with "sedentary" because most people barely move when plopped down in a chair or on a sofa. Health experts, though, have another name for it: low METs. METs stands for "metabolic equivalents," a number that represents how much energy you expend at rest versus when your body is working. (You might know the term "metabolic" in its more familiar noun form, "metabolism," which refers to how many calories you burn.) Being sedentary is defined as activity below 1.5 METs, a number you want to avoid hitting for long periods of time. What's long? By our measure, more than thirty minutes without getting up and moving around. Just by walking—and it doesn't have to be fast or involve stair climbing or oblige you to clamber up hills—you can raise your METs score threefold.

It's useful to know what METs are, but there's a much easier way to get a sense of your daily activity: keeping track of how many steps a day you take. Counting steps has become the de facto way to monitor physical activity for the simple reason that anyone can do it and it provides an accurate snapshot of how much—or how little—you move your body. There are varying accounts of how much our hunter-gatherer ancestors walked daily. Estimates run from 12,000 to 17,000 steps per day. If information about the past can be gleaned from the study of contemporary Indigenous tribes with hunter-gatherer habits, the number may be around 15,000 steps per day. Any way you look at it, most of us are falling far short of that. According to the America on the Move study (published in 2010, but we're willing to wager things haven't changed much since then, and perhaps got even worse during the COVID-19 pandemic), Americans only take an average of 5,117 steps daily (about 2.5 miles).

That's well below today's widely accepted health recommendations. By comparison, Australians average 9,695 steps daily; the Japanese, 7,168. Not coincidentally, they also have considerably lower rates of obesity. We know steps aren't the only cultural differences in our obesity rates, but it's hard to argue against more daily movement.

The more time you spend walking, the more you'll be doing to safeguard yourself from obesity, diabetes, heart disease, some cancers, osteoporosis, arthritis pain, colds and flu, depression, anxiety . . . the list goes on. And it's only part of the story. From a mobility perspective, walking moves your joints and loads your bones (including your spine and the bones in your feet—very important!) and soft tissue in ways that improve durability and protect against pain. Walking also improves aspects of health—circulation, sleep, brain chemistry—that support movement. We've paddled through raging whitewater, bombed ski runs, mountain biked down steep terrain, run on rocky trails, lifted bulky weights—but, for us, that's all extracurricular. Nothing takes the place of walking.

Assessment: Steps-Per-Day Inventory

Besides being an easy way to document activity, the great thing about counting steps is that all of them count. It's not just the steps you take when consciously going for a walk, but the "incidental" steps—non-exercise activity, or NEA—you take while, say, cruising the grocery store aisles, going up and down the stairs as you gather laundry from every room, moving from your car to a destination. Knowing that all this supplementary moving can bump up your daily numbers can be a real incentive to accumulate more of those incidental steps. Suddenly, just returning the shopping cart to the front of the store instead of just stuffing it into the space next to your car has new meaning.

We recommend that you take 8,000 to 10,000 steps per day, and 12,000 or more if at all possible. It's a reasonable amount in terms of time (we said reasonable, not easy—it's not a, um, walk in the park, and we acknowledge that—but we also think steps are imperative). Plus, it's supported by research. In 1965, the phrase "Take 10,000 steps a day" entered the health discourse, not as a result of research from the hallowed halls of American medicine, as one might expect, but from the marketing department of a Japanese company hoping to sell more pedometers. As it turns out, the pedometer manufacturer was on to something, and years of subsequent research has in fact borne out the prescient slogan. Most recently, in 2020, a large study conducted by a team of researchers from multiple national health organizations found that, compared with taking 4,000 steps per day, reaching 8,000 daily steps was associated with a 51 percent lower risk of death from all causes. Taking 12,000 steps per day was associated with a 65 percent lower risk.

In this test, we ask you to track your steps over the course of three days, then calculate your average daily distance. Given that most of us do different things on different days, you'll get a more accurate picture of how much you walk by averaging a few days' count, especially if you combine workdays with non-workdays.

WHAT IF I ALSO EXERCISE? DOES IT COUNT?

If you already walk or hike for exercise, those steps count. Likewise, runners can count their steps as well. Any other steps you take through planned physical activity (i.e., running across a squash court, dancing through a Zumba class) count, too. It's a little more challenging to translate something like swimming or cycling into a step count, and for the purposes of this assessment we suggest you ignore the time you spend engaged in any non-stepping activity.

Outside of this assessment, you can take fewer steps if you work out. For instance, if you're training several hours a day for a triathlon or are similarly engaged in truly hard exercise for long periods of time, you can choose the low end of the step count recommendation or even go somewhat below it (never skip it, though). As much as we'd like to give you a formula for converting extracurricular, non-stepping exercise into step count, there are no such magic numbers. You're going to just have to gauge it on your own. However, remember a couple of things. First, many people overestimate how much exercise they're getting, so really scrutinize how much you're moving. Second, as noted, it doesn't pay to kill it on your mountain bike or lift at the gym for three hours, only to sit for the rest of the day. You still want to move your joints and tissues in all the directions and in all the ways walking provides.

PREPARATION

To take this test, you'll need some way to count your steps. If you have a smartphone and/or smartwatch, you're set—they either have built-in step counters or will accommodate an app you can purchase to do the job. Using a fitness tracker device like a Fitbit or a simple, inexpensive clip-on pedometer are other options. If you're gadget averse, you can get a pretty good idea of your step count using this calculation: For the average person, 1 mile = 2,000 steps. The big downside of using math instead of a device is that it's going to be difficult to track the incidental steps you take during the day. Our rec: Don't cheat yourself! Spring for the $5 pedometer.

THE TEST

Beginning from the time you get up in the morning to the time you hop into bed in the evening, track your steps on three successive days. Add the three-day totals together and divide by 3 to get your average steps per day—that's your score.

WHAT YOUR RESULTS MEAN

Although we asked you to average three days' worth of steps, it's important to keep in mind that you should be getting 8,000 to 10,000 steps *every day*. You can't really bank movement. If you walk 16,000 steps on Saturday but immobilize in your Eames chair all day on Sunday (except for the short drive to pick up bagels), your tissues and joints are still going to register all that time they've spent molded into a 90-degree angle. So, whatever your steps-per-day score ends up being, remember that consistency is just as important as quantity. Get in at least 8,000 steps daily—but also don't freak out (or worse, give the whole endeavor a pass) if you can't reach that goal. *Any* steps you take are better than no steps at all.

WHEN SHOULD YOU RETEST?

Daily. That is, count your steps every day to make sure you're either advancing or continuing to hit the mark.

Walking the Walk

Consider two women. They both stand five foot six and weigh 145 pounds. One of them burns a total of 101,608 calories a year above and beyond her base calories (the number of calories she burns just in the usual course of the day). One of them burns about half that, 51,480 extra calories. Guess which one of them runs three times a week and which one of them walks 8,000 steps per day.

Of course, we've already revealed our hand—this is a chapter about steps per day, after all—so, yes, it was the 8,000-steps-a-day woman who burned the most calories. But it's still a real eye-opener to see just how big an impact staying active during the day by walking can make. Fifty-one thousand calories? You know how much ice cream that is? You couldn't eat that much ice cream, but by burning 51,000 extra calories you certainly could eat more than your friends who don't bother walking. And if you're trying to maintain or reach a healthy weight? You've got your solution right here. Multiply those extra calories burned through the years over a lifetime and they make a crazy amount of difference. For some time now we've been getting the message that people who exercise regularly are heroic, and they are—you'll never find two greater advocates of exercise than us. But let's also hear it for people who move in other ways throughout the day.

From the time in 400 BCE when Hippocrates first said, "Eating alone will not keep a man well; he must also take exercise . . . And it is necessary, as it appears, to discern the power of various exercises, both natural exercises and artificial," we've been trying to work out the formula for optimal physical activity. For much of the last sixty-five years, the focus has been on "artificial" exercise, the things we consciously do to fortify our cardiovascular system and strengthen our muscles for no other reason than to fortify our cardiovascular system and strengthen our muscles (and, for some of us, because it's fun). Most times, there's no end game when you're on a treadmill for thirty minutes or hitting HIIT (high-intensity interval training) class besides burning calories, staying healthy, and feeling good. Fair enough. These days, though, experts are looking not just at how much time you put into planned exercise, but at the precise "cocktail" of artificial and unplanned natural activity (or non-exercise activity) you achieve during a given day.

In 2021, a team of international researchers crunched the numbers from six previous studies and found that the benefits of thirty minutes of moderate-to-vigorous exercise depended on how people spent the rest of the day. If they sat for less than seven hours, their workouts reduced the odds of early death by up to 80 percent. But it did not reduce risk of premature death for people who were sedentary over eleven to twelve hours per day. As one of the researchers, Keith Diaz, PhD, professor of medicine at Columbia University, said at the time of the study's release, "It is not as simple as checking off that 'exercise' box on your to-do list. A healthy movement profile requires more than 30 minutes of daily exercise. Moving around and not remaining sedentary all day also matters."

Okay, we think we've sufficiently driven the point home: Exercise generally isn't enough. But let's get into why walking is the best solution to the activity problem. If we humans once had plenty of opportunity to move throughout the day, hunting, gathering, and doing all manner of things to stay alive, there's little need for non-exercise activity now. Unless you're in a profession that keeps you moving on your feet for long periods of time—waiting tables, kitchen work, landscaping, teaching, law enforcement, military among them—you'll likely have to plan some walks to supplement any other movement you do during the day. But we want to make the case that walking in and of itself has value beyond just helping you meet your daily steps requirement.

Better Everything

The fact that so many people have smartphones (except maybe Juliet's father, a rocket scientist who still uses a flip phone) and that every smartphone allows you to count your steps tells you that many people want to know how much they walk. You had them at "helps you live longer." Yet there is so much more you can get out of a substantial daily step count, particularly as it pertains to mobility. Walking also dovetails with so many of the other Vital Signs in this book, including those related to sleep, hip extension, and breathing. All these things intersect.

Here are the benefits of walking you can look forward to.

BETTER BODY MECHANICS (AND LESS PAIN)

Walking is the antidote to sedentariness, something we've already established is essential. But walking doesn't just get you moving; it gets you moving in the right way—that is, the way that offsets the biomechanical ills sitting perpetuates.

At its least detrimental, marathon sitting will limit your functionality, leaving your muscles and other tissues potentially stiff and tight and hampering your agility and speed. The stairs might be a slog. You may walk bent over. Forget about slipping into the bus or subway car just before the doors close; you probably won't be able to hustle fast enough to make it. That's the functional stuff. At its worst, a daily rotation from car to desk chair to La-Z-Boy will cause you pain. We talked about it earlier in the book, but it can't be said enough: Sitting adaptively shortens the musculature and connective tissues in the front of the body, from the quads to the hip flexors. Even the glutes and hamstrings adapt to sitting postures. The resulting changes can alter our abilities to move freely when we have to ultimately get out of the chair. (How has your body felt after a long flight on an airplane? Did your back feel stiff? How did your hips feel?) The good news is that walking throws a wrench into the game, taking the hips and quads and hamstrings out of the right-angle position and getting them to move in ways that nature intended. Whenever people come to us for help with chronic pain, the second thing we prescribe is walking (breathing exercises are the first—see page 70). Many of these people are athletes who think we're telling them that they now have to resign themselves to an also-ran form of exercise, walking. But that's not it at all. Even many NFL quarterbacks are now starting their training days with twenty minutes of walking.

We can't emphasize it enough: Striding, strolling, trekking, whichever way you do it—walking puts your hips into extension, lengthens tissues shortened by sitting, and puts the body back into biomechanical balance. Movement helps lubricate the joints and strengthens the muscles that support them. This can be particularly helpful if you suffer from knee pain. Unlike muscles, cartilage isn't on the blood circulation route; it receives nutrients via the movement of the joint, which helps nourishing fluid flow in and out. When you take weight on and off your knees—as well as the joints in your spine—you are bathing them in beneficial stuff. This is important even if you're not feeling pain; if you're hurting, it's imperative.

BETTER FEET

To play the long game, you must have feet that are durable and strong—essentially bombproof—and the way to get them is through loading and good sensory input. Walking provides both.

Just like the hands, the feet have receptors that respond to pressure, temperature, texture, and vibrations. They also have receptors that gather information on where the body is in space (called "proprioception"). All these receptors send sensory input to the brain, helping you balance, stay sure-footed, and make decisions that affect your movements and safety. When your feet are firing information at a rapid pace, you'll be less likely to trip and fall, twist an ankle, or contort your body in an injurious way as you try to cope with something like uneven pavement or the unexpected toy in your path. Suffice it to say that your feet are not going to get much sensory input when you're sitting. Walking, on the other hand, wakes up your feet (particularly if you do it barefoot or in flat shoes—more on this on page 121), activating the foot-to-brain system when you need to be nimble.

Something else important: Despite common use of the expression "take a load off your feet," most people in fact need to put a load *on*. There are twenty-eight bones, thirty joints, and more than one hundred muscles, tendons, and ligaments in the feet, and just like their counterparts in the rest of the body they benefit from force and contractions—it's how they adapt, remodel, and stay strong. Standing helps load the feet, but walking does it one better by adding weight and muscle contractions, both of which keep the feet flexible and supple. By walking, you're rewilding your feet, retraining them to do what they're designed for: to get you where you need to go without discomfort or pain.

BETTER CIRCULATION

If you sit in a chair and do nothing, blood will still circulate through your body. You'll also still get some benefits from the lymphatic system, another part of the circulatory system, which, to put it plainly, partly acts as the sewer of the body. Lymph, a clear fluid that flows through the lymphatic system vessels, helps clear cellular waste while also helping to maintain fluid levels and circulate immune cells that fight infection.

What we're saying is that your body doesn't completely shut down when you don't move—but it functions so much better when you do. Blood flow, of course, is propelled by the heart; get your heart to beat even a little harder—a casual stroll will do it—and it will send more nutrient- and oxygen-rich blood down the pipes. The lymphatic system is driven by muscle contractions, so the contractions your muscles make when you're walking shift the whole operation into a higher gear, flushing the debris out and decongesting the body.

You want optimal circulation in your body at all times, the reason you should walk daily. But there are also times when it's especially important. If you visit someone's hospital room shortly after they have had surgery, you may be surprised to find that the nurse has already gotten them up and walking. Movement, in this case, is critical for prompting the delivery of substances that will speed healing and the quick removal of the by-products of trauma. And you don't have to have had surgery to benefit: A boost in circulation can help even if you're just suffering from mild aches and pains. Revving up the lymphatic circulatory system in particular can also help with recovery from heavy exercise. Vigorous workouts create a lot of cellular waste that needs to be moved out of the body for the adaptations of exercise to take place.

BETTER SLEEP

A good night's sleep is a crucial element of mobility and all-around good health (more about that when you reach Vital Sign 10). And how can you get a good night's sleep? Walk. It's long been known that exercise can help tip you into a more rejuvenating slumber, but recent research looking at steps per day has shown that walking specifically also does the job. As one researcher put it, "Higher-intensity, structured exercise is not always needed to improve sleep." Take this small but interesting 2020 Hungarian study, in which two groups of sedentary people, ages nineteen to thirty-six, were enlisted. Half of them were instructed to walk 8,000 to 10,000 steps per day for four weeks, then report back on issues relating to sleep. The other group changed nothing about their activity habits. The objective of the study was to determine if walking affected sleep quality, which pertains to, among other variables, whether someone has trouble falling and staying asleep, how long they sleep, how much sleep medication they take, and how well they function during the day. The researchers also wanted to see if walking affected life satisfaction. By the end of the study, it was clear that it did—plus, the walkers had experienced improvements in all aspects of sleep quality.

A similar study, published a year earlier, had comparable results. Led by researchers at Brandeis University, the study involved a group of fifty-nine men and women, some of whom were asked to increase their steps by 2,000 a day (the intervention group) and some of whom were asked to change nothing (the control group). On days when people in the intervention group—especially women—took more steps and spent more time being active than average, they, too, reported better sleep quality and longer sleep durations.

This was not a surprise to us; we see it happen when we recommend walking as a sleep aid to the people we work with. When members of elite military forces are having trouble sleeping, they're prescribed step counters and daily accumulations of 10,000 to 15,000 steps. The most obvious explanation for the better sleep effect is that walking tires you out. But there may be other reasons as well. Walking, like other forms of physical activity, affects various chemicals in the body, ranging from cell-signaling proteins to brain neurotransmitters, that researchers suspect may enhance sleep. The truth is, they're still trying to figure it out, but there are a few things that seem clear.

One of them is that physical activity lowers levels of depression and anxiety, conditions that can prevent and disrupt sleep. In particular, 200 minutes of walking a week (that's about a half hour a day—much less than 8,000 steps!) has been associated with fewer symptoms of depression. (Sitting more than seven hours a day, on the other hand, has been associated with more depressive symptoms.) Walking's calming effects also help to lower the anxiety that keeps people up at night. Even a little walking has been shown to quiet the mind. And if that walking is done outside during daylight, there can be additional benefits. Exposure to sunlight, especially morning light, shifts forward the time you get sleepy, making it more likely that you won't burn the midnight oil, will go to bed at a reasonable time, and thus will get in all the hours of shut-eye you need. (For this same reason, going for a walk when you arrive in a foreign place can help you adjust to a new time zone and reduce jet lag.)

BETTER BRAIN FUNCTION

It's a truth universally—if erroneously—acknowledged that a person tied to their desk for hours will be more productive than the office gadabout. We say "erroneously" because it turns out that office workers who sit for periods as long as four hours have less blood flow to their brains, a drop that can potentially result in hazy thinking and diminished memory. This discovery was made at the Research Institute for Sport and Exercise Sciences at Liverpool John Moores University, where researchers measured brain blood flow in fifteen workers after three different scenarios: four hours of uninterrupted sitting; four hours of sitting interrupted every thirty minutes with two-minute walks; and four hours of sitting interrupted every two hours with eight-minute walks. The more frequent walking breaks were the winners, offsetting the drop in workers' blood flow more than either continuous sitting or walking every two hours. (The researchers didn't look at workers who were using standing desks, but research shows that standing enhances focus and memory—more on this in Vital Sign 9. So imagine if you're standing during work *and* taking walking breaks. The potential double-whammy brain boost is exciting!)

The beauty of walking, though, is not just that it curtails the decline in blood coursing through the brain. Done with even a small amount of vigor and at a reasonable length (ten minutes even), it *increases* the flow, also raising a tide of neurochemicals that similarly benefit the brain. One of those chemicals is serotonin, the feel-good hormone that may have something to do with why physical activity improves mood and decreases depression. Another is a molecule called "brain-derived neurotrophic factor" (BDNF), which helps brain cells function fully and even grow. One of the best ways to trigger neuroplasticity is to walk fast. The brain senses the activity and, to adapt, grows new connections that improve cognitive ability and strengthen areas subject to age-related decline. It can even help an unfocused mind become more attentive. For all these reasons, Harvard psychiatrist John Ratey, MD, author of *Spark: The Revolutionary New Science of Exercise and the Brain,* has variously called physical activity "a little bit of Prozac and a little bit of Ritalin" and "Miracle-Gro" for the brain.

Several studies have also found that physical activity enhances creativity. One Stanford University study even found that walking in particular—whether done on a treadmill facing a blank wall or on a verdant towpath along a rumbling river—helped people become an average of 60 percent more creative than when they spent the same amount of time sitting. And all it took was ten minutes. The researchers tested innovative thinking using various tests, including one that asked the study participants to come up with alternative ways to use common objects and another that asked them to come up with analogies for different phrases.

If you've ever tried solving a problem to no avail, only to have the answer come to you while you're walking your dog, this research will likely come as no surprise. Visual artists, writers, and musicians use physical activity to jump-start their brains all the time. Walking won't make you the next Toni Morrison or Pablo Picasso, but it seems certain that it can help boost your mental productivity and, perhaps most important, deflect some of the adverse changes to the brain that come with age. We can say from personal experience that walking is a good time to problem solve. Solutions seem to come more readily when we're walking quietly, alone with our thoughts. We don't always walk this way. We walk and talk with friends, listen to books, podcasts, and music—it's a great way to multitask, and if it doesn't provide the silence needed for creative thought, well, it provides a brain boost of another sort: information intake.

It can also help you deal with pain. You know those endorphins—aka runner's high—you're always hearing about? Those brain chemicals, known as the "endogenous opioid system" and activated by movement, are the body's natural medicine, our do-it-yourself way of relieving pain. You don't have to be a runner to get endorphins flowing, but some evidence suggests that the more walking you do (one of the reasons we recommend you walk daily), the likelier you are to have a higher tolerance for pain. Neuroscientists at Duquesne University discovered this when they had women walk three, five, and ten times during a weeklong study. Each bout was thirty minutes, walked at a moderate pace. The researchers then tested the women's pain perception when subjected to heat and pressure. Those who walked five and ten times a week (but not three) found the test 60 percent less painful after walking than they did at the start of the study.

YOUR BRAIN ON PHYSICAL ACTIVITY

Cognitive Effects of Exercise in Preadolescent Children
Average composite of 20 students' brains taking the same test after sitting quietly or taking a 20-minute walk

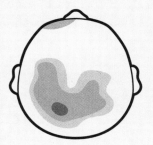

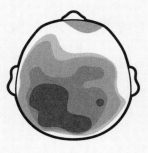

BRAIN AFTER SITTING QUIETLY   BRAIN AFTER 20-MINUTE WALK

Source: Derived from research by Dr. C. H. Hillman, University of Illinois Urbana–Champaign (2009).

BETTER STRESS CONTROL

In our line of work, we get the chance to meet some interesting people, and one of them is Joyce Shulman, who created (with her husband, Eric) a company called 99 Walks (99walks.fit). With regular walking challenges and classes and an app that virtually connects walkers around the world, the company is devoted to encouraging people to get out (or even stay in on a treadmill) and walk. All this is to say that Joyce has had the opportunity to see into the hearts and minds of a lot of walkers. So when we asked her what she heard most often about walking's benefits, she was quick with an answer: less stress. "Most of our walkers report that walking has a positive impact on their mood," says Joyce, who herself found that getting out and walking after the difficult delivery of her first child made her feel human again.

There are likely a lot of reasons for this (see box on page 117), including the aforementioned (page 112) correlation between physical activity and lower levels of depression and anxiety. Walking, like other forms of movement, also has an effect on stress hormones. Produced in the adrenal glands, these hormones, cortisol and adrenaline, are what helps the body shift into fight-or-flight mode when encountering danger (say, a lion, or a roaring boss, or perhaps the beastly chaos of a bad day). If you're feeling stressed out, levels of cortisol and adrenaline in your blood will be high. But if you engage in some moderate physical activity, like a nice long walk, levels of those hormones will drop and you'll likely feel better. The endorphins kicking in will lift your mood, too.

STEPS, COMMUNITY, AND LESS LONELINESS

When our girls were in elementary school, we had a revelation. We'd been doing what most parents were doing: packing our kids into the car, battling the traffic, waiting in the drop-off line, quickly rolling the kids out of the car when we finally reached the head of the line, pulling back into the traffic to get to work, and feeling frazzled. Everyone, kids included, was frazzled.

So we decided to take a different tack. We made a plan to get up twenty minutes earlier and start walking our girls to school. Our older daughter was in third grade and our youngest was in kindergarten. Both were able to do the mile-and-a-half distance, and it turned into a lovely family time. We'd walk and talk, nobody on a phone, and saunter through a field where we'd look at bugs and leaves. Despite the fact that the girls attended a community school—most everyone attending lived within a two-mile range—we rarely saw any other kids walking or biking on our route.

We'd been walking for about a year when we heard about something called the Walking School Bus (walkingschoolbus.org). It's a protocol, recommended by the U.S. Department of Transportation, for gathering a group of children together to walk to school, a sort of "bus" with a driver (one or more adults) that bypasses the morning rush and provides a safe way for everyone to get in some exercise. We were already making the trek, so why not get some other kids, and hopefully parents, involved? We put up a flyer and made an announcement at school saying, "Every morning at 7:50 we will be standing on the corner of X and Y, and we will be happy to walk your kids to school. Rain or shine." We ended up getting ten to fifteen kids in the beginning, then it grew to forty or fifty (the numbers ebbed and flowed). Other parents began signing up as "drivers," too, and over the course of the eight years our girls were at the school, new friendships were born among both parents and kids in various grades who might not otherwise have had a chance to meet.

The Walking School Bus fostered a great sense of community, freed the parents from some of the morning hassle, was healthy for everyone (one mom lost ten pounds), and was fun, even in inclement weather. What we realized, too, was that with the round-trip walk, we had already accumulated about 5,000 steps by approximately 8:30 a.m. Here was proof that even if you have a crazy schedule, replacing driving or public transportation with walking whenever possible can get you well on your way to the 8,000 to 10,000 steps-per-day mark. All the better if you can do it in a way that fosters time with family and friends.

While the Walking School Bus is a great solution for people with young kids, you don't have to be an elementary school parent to be part of a walking community. And if you need some incentive to do it, consider that the social benefits can be invaluable. Joyce Shulman's 99 Walks did a survey of 2,300 women walkers connected via its app, and 73 percent of them said they sometimes felt lonely. Feeling disconnected isn't just sad; good research suggests it can shorten your lifespan. But Joyce's survey also found that women who walk regularly with friends are two and a half times less likely to experience loneliness—just one more reason to seek out others to walk with. "I run a company, I'm a mother, and always have 101 things to do—I'm one of 'those' people who are super busy," says Joyce. "But walking with my 'pack' ticks off a lot of boxes for me. I get exercise, I get to spend time in nature, it gives me time for myself, and it lets me connect with friends. Four things in one."

Physical Practice: Intentional Walks and More-Steps Strategies

In some ways, we doubt you need any instructions on how to accomplish this physical practice: Just move your feet and go until you've managed to get 8,000 to 10,000 steps a day (some of them incidental, but some undoubtedly from pointedly going for a walk). But because walking also gives you the opportunity to incorporate other practices into your daily step count, this physical practice includes instructions on how to do a Nose-Breathing Walk and, if you're up for it, some rucking (carrying objects while you walk). Plus, some people actually do need a little guidance on the particulars of walking. If that's you, here's what we need you to know.

DON'T WORRY ABOUT THE TIMING OR DURATIONS OF YOUR WALKS—We have one rule about timing and duration of walks, and that is: There are no rules. Just get your steps in. There may be some advantages to walking in the morning. If everyone woke up and went for a walk in the morning, chances are they'd feel more alert, ready to face the day. Getting exposure to morning sun can also help you sleep better. We think you're going to have more success if you ask yourself when you have the time to walk instead of trying to adhere to some idea that the "best" time to walk is morning or some other time. As to the duration of your walks, you will probably need to go on some longer walks to reach the 8,000 to 10,000 a day mark, but again, do whatever it takes to hit the goal. If walking briskly to burn more calories or as a cardiovascular exercise, then, yes, getting your heart rate up for at least twenty minutes is a good target to shoot for. Likewise, if your goal is to improve your endurance, longer (and faster) can be better. We are all for challenging yourself. But you don't have to get your heart rate up substantially or walk for any particular length of time to meet the steps-per-day objective.

CHECK YOUR FOOT POSITION—For the best organization of your body—meaning that everything is aligned and there are no imbalances putting undue pressure on your back or other body parts—all you need to do is walk with your feet pointing straight ahead. You have a greater chance of doing so if you start in what's called the "reference foot position." In this neutral position, as you are standing comfortably with your feet straight and underneath your hips, you should have 50 percent of your weight on the balls of your feet and 50 percent of your weight on the heels. Also, if you look down, your ankles should be in the middle of your feet, not collapsing in, out, toward the front, or toward the back. If your ankles lean one way or the other or your knees knock in, see if you can't find that middle position. It would be crazy to think that you're going to check the position of your feet every time you walk, but if you do check in periodically to make sure you're standing in the reference foot position, you can begin to train your brain for better locomotion.

While they may seem fairly inert, there is a ton of motion happening in your feet when you walk. Making an effort to walk with your feet straight allows you to tap into your natural

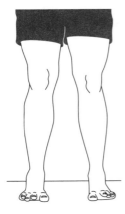 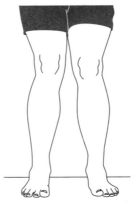 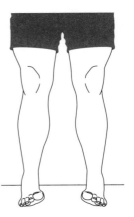

| Balanced: Ankles in the middle. | Ankles too far to the inside. | Ankles too far to the outside. |

mechanics and put more power into your walk. Imagining that you're walking on either side of a narrow line can help, too. Eventually, reference foot position will become a habit and your walking stance will improve.

CONSIDER YOUR SHOES (OR LACK THEREOF)

Stand in the reference foot position and notice how it feels. Now put on the shoes you usually walk in. What kind of input are you getting? Are you still in the reference foot position? Balanced on your feet, 50 percent on the heels, 50 percent on the balls? Or are your shoes guiding you one way or the other? Are your toes squished?

Most people are walking around in ridiculously pillowed or high-heeled shoes that not only knock their feet out of alignment but also make it more difficult for the brain to get the all-important sensory input from the feet. To our mind, the more you can do barefoot, the better. Provided that you're not working out in a place with sharp elements on the ground, it's safe and even healthy for you to walk, lift weights, or do any other activity without shoes (some activities like cycling and perhaps trail running will obviously require shoes).

As for what to wear when you do wear shoes, we are passionate advocates of choosing the flattest shoes possible, or, as we think of them, shoes that disrupt the feet the least. Think about how your feet are built. They're made with the heel and ball of the foot in the same plane to afford you the best balance. This is not a call for you to go out and get new shoes for walking or working out, but rather to wear shoes the rest of the time that have only as much padding as needed to protect your feet from the elements. When it's time to get new shoes, then, yes, go for a more minimalist shoe. When you try them on, give yourself the reference foot position test before handing over your credit card.

Consider, too, that arch support is not something you generally need to worry about. Again, this goes back to the basic physiology of the feet. The arch is a nonloading surface; it's not meant to bear weight (the balls and heels of the feet are) but rather to be springy, to put a spring in your step. We've asked rooms full of people to remove their shoes, and when we get them into the reference foot position, everyone—even those with the flattest feet—can create some kind of arch as they stand without any arch support aid. (We'll talk more about your feet in Vital Sign 8.)

Some people, we know, are devoted to high heels, and we get it. Just take them off when you get home from work or a night out. In other words, wear them as little as possible. The imbalance created by heels has the potential to stress the Achilles tendons and the calf muscles and can even exacerbate conditions you might not expect. We have a friend who has very bad pelvic floor dysfunction, which can cause urine leakage when you move or sneeze. She's also five foot two and an executive who feels naked without high heels; it's part of her identity. But during the pandemic, when she was working from home, she switched to wearing flat tennis shoes and it made a big difference in her pelvic floor dysfunction symptoms. Ordinarily, you wouldn't connect the two—heels and a urine leakage—but it just goes to show how much your feet affect the whole of your body.

In that same vein: flip-flops? Hard pass. Kelly has posted some semi-controversial things on Instagram (stop icing injuries is one of them—see page 190), but those things don't hold a candle to the times he's told people not to wear flip-flops. Let's just say it's not a popular opinion. Here's the thing. If you're wearing flip-flops to the pool or beach or to protect your feet in a gas station, fine. But if you're walking any distance in them, you will feel the consequences. Flip-flops don't allow the big toe to flex, which allows the foot to push off the ground. So the body compensates, hyperstiffening the plantar fascia (tissue connecting the heel bone to the toes) and ankle, which can cause pain down the line. Slides present the same problem. Make sure the shoes you're walking in have a back.

THREE WALKS

As noted earlier, walking fast has its rewards in terms of calories burned and cardiovascular benefits. We're all for it. Yet the main thing is to just walk, no matter if you prefer to stroll or race down your chosen path. Here are a few ways to do it.

1. Nose-Breathing Walk

This walk allows you to work on your CO_2 tolerance (see page 53) as you get your daily steps in. It can be done for any duration of time. You may want to do the breathing part for only a portion of your walk, which is fine, too. Just try to work up to doing it for the entire time.

As you begin your walk, breathing through your nose only, take the longest, slowest inhale you can take, about ten seconds. Hold the breath for as long as you can as you continue walking, then exhale slowly through your nose. Repeat every one to two minutes depending on your tolerance.

2. Thrice Daily Walks

If you're someone who is usually pressed for time, you can still likely spare ten minutes. Rather than trying to work in a long walk each day, simply break it up: Walk for ten minutes after each meal.

3. Barefoot Walks

Walking barefoot hasn't really been popular since hippies roamed the earth in the '60s and '70s, but we're hoping for a comeback. Going shoeless gives your feet lots of sensory input, strengthens them, and helps you avoid the toll shoes can take on the heel cords, arches, and other structures in the feet. If it's safe—meaning you can travel in an area free of glass and other sharp debris—we recommend doing one barefoot walk a week, or at least a couple of laps around the block. If it's not possible, go barefoot as much as possible as you walk around the house and your backyard. You might even designate a day for it—Barefoot Saturday.

EXTRA CREDIT: RUCKING

The science of how our modern human body evolved is itself ever evolving. And yet, anthropologists are pretty sure that we became upright walkers because it was more energy efficient than hunting for food on all fours. Helping to bolster this theory is the fact that chimpanzees, placed on a treadmill, required 75 percent more energy to walk than upright humans. It's just easier to walk on two feet.

Another, adjacent theory is that biped walking evolved to allow us to carry things. We are, in other words, built to move *and* to lug things from place to place. Carrying is a human trait, and aside from how it improved our lives—being able to carry sustenance, tools, even people as needed—it also provided a way for us to safely load our spines and our feet. Maybe when you think about "loading" your mind automatically draws a picture of someone in a gym doing biceps curls with dumbbells. But loading is really just adding weight, any weight, to a body part in order to make it stronger, and it does not have to be achieved through formalized resistance training.

With that in mind, let us introduce you to rucking. If you don't already know about it, rucking is carrying weight in a backpack while you walk (the name comes from the military term for backpack, "rucksack"), and it's an elegant, efficient way to increase the impact of your steps per day. For some people, rucking has also become a substitute for running. Our observation is that when you're in your twenties, everyone can run without much problem. But then there's a precipitous drop-off, and by the time you're in your forties you have about one friend who can run more than five miles and feel good. The rest of them are injured or don't like the way running feels anymore. That's when we see a lot of them take up rucking as a lower-impact way to an equivalent amount of exercise.

In some ways, you may already be rucking. Wearing a backpack and carrying a briefcase or a sizable purse are all forms of rucking. (While we're on the topic, we recommend backpacks or crossbody bags for functional wear because they distribute the load across the body. Switch one-arm bags frequently to get some of the same effect.) The easiest way to add the rucking effect to your physical practice is to throw a few household items—say, a few cans, some books, or a sack of flour—into a backpack, strap it on, and go for your usual walk. You can also ruck without the rucksack. Joe de Sena, the founder of the Spartan Race, a competition involving obstacles, famously carries around a 44-pound kettlebell weight everywhere he goes. The two of us sometimes carry a 30-pound sandbag when we walk, and we always make the choice to carry things when the opportunity arises. For instance, when we travel, we opt for duffel bags instead of rolling suitcases so that we have to carry our luggage. (We knew we made the right choice when we were in Thailand and saw other travelers struggling to pull their rolling bags across a beach.) There is also gear made specifically for rucking. GORUCK, a company run by Jason McCarthy, a former member of the U.S. Army Special Forces, and his wife, Emily McCarthy, formerly of the CIA, sells backpacks with pockets for weighted plates and other related equipment. What Jason McCarthy has had to say about rucking sums it up pretty nicely: "It's strength and cardio in one. It's cardio for the person who hates running, and strength work for the person who hates lifting."

Nine Strategies for Walking More

- Walk while you talk. Use personal phone calls and even work meeting calls as opportunity to walk, whether it's outside or just around your home or office space.
- Communicate in person. At work, walk to talk to a colleague before you call or click.
- Walk your dog! If you don't have one, maybe this will inspire you to get one: A U.K. study found that dog-owners walk twenty-two minutes more per day than non-dog-owners. At the very least, borrow your neighbor's dog—it's the rare canine that won't enjoy an extra outing.
- Walk your kid to school. If it's safe, there is no better way to get steps in while also doing something healthy for your child (see Steps, Community, and Less Loneliness, page 117).

- Take the stairs. Okay, you've heard this one before, but we'd be remiss if we didn't remind you that taking the stairs is another way to get steps in without having to go for a formal walk. Every flight counts.
- Shop in person. During the pandemic, a lot of us got used to ordering groceries and just about everything else online. Wander the aisles in person, however, and you're going to move way more than you would by letting your fingers do the walking on your keyboard.
- Park far from your destination or get off public transportation early. There's no rule that says you have to be delivered to the doorstep of where you're going; that's just something most of us have gotten used to. Break the habit. You may not be able to walk the whole way to your destination, but it doesn't mean you can't get some steps in.
- Use wait time to walk. If you're taking someone to the doctor or dentist, don't just hang out in the waiting room. Take the time to walk. Likewise, if you're at your kid's volleyball tournament and there's downtime (and there almost always is), walk around the venue a few times. If you have to wait for a table at a restaurant, give them your cell and tell them to call you when your table is ready (a lot of restaurants do this now anyway) while you walk around the block.
- Walk around your house. We've heard about people, stymied by bad weather or poor air quality, who've set up obstacle courses in their homes just to get more steps in. Sure, you're not going to rack up the miles, but it's better than nothing. Or consider a treadmill. Al Roker, the *Today Show* weatherman, vowed to walk more after a prostate cancer diagnosis. To avoid New York City's cold temps (and who better than a weatherman to know when to stay inside?), Al took to walking in place—a very good idea.

FUTURE-PROOF
YOUR NECK AND SHOULDERS

ASSESSMENT **PART 1: Airport Scanner Arms-Raise Test;
PART 2: Shoulder Rotation Test**

PHYSICAL PRACTICE **Shoulder Flexion, Upper Back,
and Rotator Cuff Mobilizations**

REMEMBER THE AIRPORT security full-body scanner we talked about in Vital Sign 3? Let's head back over to the TSA station to see what else we can learn about the body. This time, though, instead of focusing on the lower body, we're interested in the upper body and, more specifically, the neck and shoulders.

Many a time, as we've watched people assume the required arms-above-the-head stance, we've seen them contort their neck and other body parts just to get their arms up for those few required seconds. Their body is solving the problem—maybe they overextend their neck or banana their back—but it's nonetheless very difficult for them to get, let alone hold, their arms aloft for any significant amount of time. And that's a clue that something is missing: namely, complete range of motion in the shoulders.

The shoulders and their adjacent body parts, the neck and the thoracic spine (also known as the "T-spine" or upper back), are not something people think about much—until they hurt or you realize you can't do something you thought you could. Like throwing a ball for your dog, picking up a kid and placing them on your shoulders, swimming laps freestyle, putting away linens on a high shelf, lifting a suitcase into the overhead compartment, and, yes, raising your arms for the airport scanner. If you can't perform these basic moves, it may also make it unlikely that you'll be able to pick up new activities that require reaching or raising your arms. Say you want to try swimming, weight training, or mastering a pull-up; it may be difficult. Say you want to paint your bedroom. Even painting on canvas, depending on how you do it, can be nearly impossible if you can't get your arms up for long. Worst-case scenario (but not out of the realm of possibility) is that, as you grow older, even things like pulling a sweater over your head or washing your hair will cause you discomfort because your shoulders have such a limited range of motion. But give your shoulders the movement they need to stay supple, and you can do pull-ups or repaint the walls of your home to your heart's content.

You may have noticed that all those things we mentioned above are probably not things you do every day. We don't throw spears any longer, nor carry things overhead or climb trees like our ancestors. Unless you're a swimmer or do certain exercises that require raising the arms (pressing overhead, for instance), most people's shoulders get just about zero input. There's a reason that downward dog is a central feature in the ancient system of yoga. It's a long-held notion that we need to get our arms up and our shoulders working; otherwise, they're only subject to the potential rounding forward that comes from sitting most of the day.

The neck doesn't get much input, either. Think about how often you look straight ahead into the glare of a computer or television screen. If your car has a backup camera, you don't even have to look over your shoulder to go in reverse or parallel park anymore. Perhaps you bend your neck and hunch your back to look at your phone or laptop all day. At least looking down gets you to move your neck a bit. But as with anything, overdoing it has consequences (it even has a name: "text neck"). For the most part, though, few people turn their heads nearly enough, and when they do, they notice that it hurts.

Neck pain can have many causes. There are the aforementioned tech-driven positions. Your neck could hurt because you're not breathing efficiently, or because you're worried about your kid getting into college and you're grinding your teeth at night, or because your spouse is a pain in the ass and the stress is causing you to neck breathe (see page 62). But shoulder dysfunction often plays a role in or exacerbates neck pain. As we've pointed out before, everything is connected—the body is a system of interlocking pieces—and the neck and shoulders in particular are a couplet. So, when someone comes to us with neck pain, we automatically look into their shoulder range of motion, both as the potential cause of the pain and as the solution.

The body is always in flux, your range of motion a living, breathing entity. Go ahead and have a baby and watch how things change (and change back). Run a marathon, then fly home on an overnight flight and see how your range of motion can contract. Spend two brutal years grinding out papers in grad school and at the end you'll notice, "Wow, I have a different body than I had before." If you understand this, you can understand how it's possible to restore normal movement to body parts that have been in the dry docks. And this includes the shoulders.

We are the first to tell you that the shoulders and neck are complex and that there are many different issues that can crop up. There are people who specialize in shoulder rehab at the Olympic level, as well as shoulder specialists who focus solely on the shoulder and neck grievances of Major League Baseball players. With age, conditions like rotator cuff injuries and frozen shoulder crop up—in China and Japan this sort of "gluing" in the shoulder socket is called "fifty-year-old shoulder"—but we're not addressing those limiting factors here. Instead, this Vital Sign is designed to introduce you to the basic workings of the shoulder area so that, through simple movements, you can have full access to all the positions the shoulder is capable of. Those movements may help you avoid shoulder injury and pain, but they're not necessarily the cure. Here, our aim is to get you thinking not about what your shoulders can't do, but what they're *supposed* to do. That's going to affect the immediate area, neck included, and make your whole body work better, as well as help you avoid neck and shoulder problems altogether.

WHY YOU'RE DOING THIS

This is a public service message for you—from Germany. A few years ago, the pharmacy chain DocMorris ran an ad that perfectly sums up our philosophy.

It begins with an older gentleman getting out of bed before sunrise and looking forlornly at photos of his family. Still dressed in his pajamas and robe, he stumbles out to a storage room, where he finds an old kettlebell. He can barely lift it. Day after day, the man rises early and practices lifting the kettlebell, ignoring the nosy neighbor clearly alarmed at his efforts. Gradually, he's able to raise the kettlebell higher and higher. As the ad nears its end, the old gent dresses up, wraps a gift, and drives to his daughter's home for a Christmas celebration. His young granddaughter opens the gift, a big, bright star for the Christmas tree. He then picks the girl up and raises her high enough to place it on top of the tall tree. The tagline is: "So you can take care of what matters in life." We cried, of course.

We live in a world where it's easy to lose perspective on why we should be fit. To look better? To satisfy our competitive urges? Nothing wrong with either of those incentives. But when it comes down to brass tacks, there's no better reason than to be strong and healthy for yourself and for those you love and who love you. Remember this on those days you wake up feeling like you don't want to work on shoulder rotation or go for a walk; it may help you get out of bed.

Assessment: Part 1: Airport Scanner Arms-Raise Test; Part 2: Shoulder Rotation Test

The assessments in this chapter are designed to look at two particular elements of shoulder mobility. The first one looks at shoulder flexion. That is, when asked to raise your arms overhead and move them behind you, how far can they go? How close to the end range—the farthest point in their natural range—can you get? The second test appraises the external (outward from the body) rotation of your shoulders. Again, can you get to the farthest point that your shoulders can roll back?

At first glance, you might think these are simply measures of how naturally flexible you are. But remember: We are assessing your ability to access baseline ranges of motion, NOT your ability to perform superhero gymnast moves. With both of these assessments, the goal is to see what your current ranges of motion are, as well as to see how well you can use them.

PART 1: AIRPORT SCANNER ARMS-RAISE TEST

We named this test after the most revealing (and public) place to observe people's shoulder mobility. The test is a little more elaborate than simply raising your arms above your head, but still very straightforward.

PREPARATION

The ideal aid for doing this test is a piece of PVC pipe a couple of feet long. If you don't have one, a lightweight broomstick or some other light, pole-like object will do. If you don't have any of the above, use a rolled-up dish towel or do the test without anything in your hands.

THE TEST

Lie facedown on the floor with your arms extended straight in front of you, hands holding a piece of PVC pipe. Point your thumbs toward the ceiling and allow the pipe to rest in the crook between your thumbs and forefingers. Keeping your forehead and belly in contact with the floor, arms straight (parallel) and thumbs up, lift your arms up as high as they'll go. Hold for five inhales and exhales. Avoid holding your breath or bending your elbows.

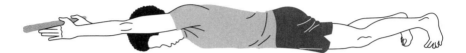

You may find this more difficult if you ever had a grandparent who told you to sit up straight at the table.

WHAT YOUR RESULTS MEAN

How did that feel? Just taking the test can make you aware of how much tension you hold in your shoulders.

Can't lift your arms—You are way below where you should be, perhaps because you rarely have occasion to raise your arms overhead. The good news is that the physical practices should help you improve quickly if you do them daily.

Can lift off the floor but can't sustain or do it while breathing—Let this small amount of movement encourage you—there's plenty more where that came from if you do the work to access it.

1 to 2 inches off the floor—This is a sign that you can access the position, but you don't own it yet. With a little fatigue, you may not be able to hold it long. The physical practice will help you improve not only range of motion but stamina as well.

2+ inches off the floor—Awesome. Lack of shoulder flexion is not your problem. You may not need to do the Wall Hang (page 144) every day, but it should still be part of your repertoire to maintain that flexion.

WHEN SHOULD YOU RETEST?
Once a week.

PART 2: SHOULDER ROTATION TEST
Unlike the previous test, this test can't be measured in inches; it calls for a more subjective reading. What you'll be doing is placing your arms on the floor and assessing how much force you're able to press down with. Don't let the word "force" trip you up if the last time you picked up a weight was in high school gym class and don't consider yourself very strong. The test is not a measure of strength, but rather a gauge of whether the amount of rotation you have allows you to generate power. Most humans are born with the strength they need to do daily activities, yet that strength doesn't only rely on muscle. It also depends on how well your joints allow you to move (a biceps, bulging or not, isn't going to move itself). So even if you don't think you need power, you do—it's all just a matter of degree. That's why everyone from desk jockeys to professional athletes need to pay attention to mobility. Here, specifically, having a more functional rotator cuff will translate into MUCH better shoulder efficiency, stability, and durability.

PREPARATION
You won't need anything for this test, just some clear floor space. Have your wrists free of a watch or any jewelry.

THE TEST
Lie faceup on the floor, knees bent, feet flat on the floor. Place your arms out to the side and bend your elbows at a 90-degree angle, palms facing up. Now, by rolling your shoulders back in their sockets (this is a subtle move), see how hard you can push the backs of your wrists and hands down into the floor. Continue pushing for five inhales and exhales. Avoid holding your breath.

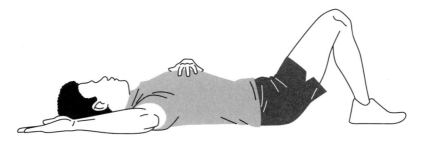

Each shoulder's rotator cuff should be able to fully rotate, and powerfully.

WHAT YOUR RESULTS MEAN

There's no scoring for this one. Just have a sense of how much force you were able to generate so that you can compare it to your power after doing the mobilizations.

WHEN SHOULD YOU RETEST?

We suggest redoing the Shoulder Rotation Test immediately after the first time you do the Rotator Cuff Mobilization, because it has such a dramatic impact on rotation. After that, give yourself a week of doing the physical practice, then try the tests again. Test once more after another week. After that, retest as you see fit to check whether you've improved.

The Octopus and the Great Big C

You know where the shoulders are. You know that some people have broad ones, other people have sloped ones, and that they once, in the 1980s, were host (some would say regrettably) to a fashionable trend known as shoulder pads. But do you know how the shoulders really work? It will help you understand why they matter so much in relation to the rest of the body if you do.

The shoulders consist primarily of large, somewhat triangular bones that lie flat across the upper back and attach to the collarbones. These bones, otherwise known as the shoulder blades or scapulae, have a socket on one side where the top of the arm (a ball-like structure called the "humerus") attaches.

Also included in this construction is the rotator cuff, a web of muscles and connective tissues that provide support and allow the arm and shoulder to move. Now visualize this: Your rotator cuff is like an octopus that has swum, headfirst, into a seashell. That seashell is your shoulder blade. And from within that shoulder blade, this octopus rotator cuff reaches out its "arms" to steer, guide, position, organize, stabilize, and rotate the humerus. That's how your arms are able to do what they need to do.

One of the problems with modern posture is that, because so many of us work at a computer for hours, our shoulders slouch forward and our upper back rounds. We become C-shaped organisms. This disrupts the octopus-seashell relationship, because now the shell is being pulled forward as the body assumes this habitual C posture, and that knocks the octopus–rotator cuff off its game. Suddenly, the octopus's arms no longer have a balanced grasp on the humerus. Some of the arms are stretched out super long, some are compressed. When you go to raise *your* arms (or do any of the other things that arms are called on to do), this disruption is going to take away some functioning. To see what we mean, hunch your shoulders forward and raise one arm. Then get into a position where you can take your biggest breath (this will undoubtedly mean you'll be uncurling the C) and raise your arm again. Feel the difference? When you're out of C position, the octopus–rotator cuff is a lot better at its job.

The C position is not merely the curse of the deskbound. Sometimes you need to be in a C for sports, but most times you don't. You shouldn't, for instance, be in a rounded position when doing strength-training rows. On the water, paddlers and rowers with good technique will have an upright posture not only because it allows them to generate more power, but also because it helps them avoid injury. In the past we've seen rowers with broken ribs, fractured because, by curling inward, their muscles were pulling on their ribs. So whatever you do during your day, try to avoid the C position as much as you can.

(Just as an aside here, there's an old maxim that goes, "The hands are clever." This suggests that, even if you end up with the most restricted rotator cuff and worst shoulder range of motion, with little ability to raise your arms, nature won't let you go hungry. Your survival instinct will kick in and you'll just feed yourself by bringing your face to your hands. The amazing dexterity of your hands and forearms can hide a lot of missing shoulder range of motion. Poor shoulder range of motion may actually be one of the root causes of golf and tennis elbow, but it escapes notice for a while because the hands and forearms compensate. We also see this type of compensation when we watch a baking show where one of the judges always bends over to taste the cakes. We suspect that she has shoulder trouble!)

There is more to the shoulder story. The shoulder blades also attach to the trapezius muscles. Known more familiarly as the "traps," these muscles extend from the base of the head/top of the neck, across the shoulder blades, and halfway down the back. They even have attachments to your collarbones. Among other things, the traps help you shrug and move your head side to side. If you take your shoulder blades and spin them forward, called "protraction," your traps get very busy trying to hold up your neck. Do it for long enough and those muscles get overworked. Once again, another part of the shoulder area architecture is thrown off, creating an imbalance where one structure is doing more than its share of the work. No wonder we start to see error signals like tightness, discomfort, and pain in the shoulders and neck. We start to see loss of function, too.

So now that the neck has entered the picture, there is something else to consider. One is your head. When your body is well organized and your head is perfectly balanced on your neck, you don't really register it as a burden. In this regard, you're strong. Even babies at a certain point can hold their little heads up. But say you are constantly looking down at your phone or your body is in the rounded C position, causing your head to jut forward. For every inch forward it goes, your head adds a 10-pound load to your neck. In response, the traps and other muscles and connective tissue around the shoulders and around the upper spine start to get stiff because it's easier for your body to hold your heavy head up in that rigid, locked position. The body in all its wisdom will do what it has to do to solve a technical problem, but there are usually repercussions of a functional nature. Try to look over your shoulder with your head projecting forward and you'll see that you can't look very far.

UP IN ARMS: A PERSONAL STORY

In early 2019, I, Juliet, raised my arms overhead and considered it one of my greatest physical accomplishments, right up there with winning the whitewater world championships and giving birth to two children. What made it so significant was that, about a month earlier, I had had breast reconstruction surgery; two weeks before that I had had a double mastectomy. Six weeks after the final surgery I was able to raise my arms so completely that I could do a pull-up (I started with hanging first). Never have I been so grateful for the range of motion in my shoulders.

I was diagnosed with Stage 1A breast cancer at the very end of 2018. I'd had some lumps and bumps before, so my physician had already been watching my breast health for about ten years. This particular problem was discovered through a routine ob-gyn exam. My cancer was very treatable, requiring surgery, but not chemotherapy or radiation. In that regard, I felt fortunate. But like every person who has cancer, I had to ask, Why? I had a panel of genetic tests that showed I had no inherited risk of the disease. A lot of people think that it's just the *BRCA* genes that increase your susceptibility to breast cancer; in fact, there are about 110 genes that can contribute to a risk of the disease. I was also tested for a genetic predisposition to other cancers, and those tests came back negative as well. So how did I get breast cancer? Probably environmental factors, but I'll never know for sure.

I decided to have the double mastectomy and a reconstruction because of the strange history with my breasts and the chance the cancer could recur. It was decided that, because I was fit and healthy, I could do the two surgeries almost back-to-back. I went in on a Monday for the mastectomy, then went back two weeks later for the reconstruction. The surgery has even evolved since then. A friend had breast cancer a few years later and did the two surgeries all at once. But no matter how you do it, it's still two major surgeries, both physically and emotionally taxing.

One of the side effects of having these two operations so close together is that you can potentially lose some vital mobility, especially in your arms. It becomes very difficult to raise them overhead. I had another friend who'd also had a mastectomy and reconstruction, and she still couldn't lift her arms nine months down the line. I was determined not to get to that point. (My friend was able to regain mobility over time, but it took a lot of work.) Although this isn't really a shoulder mobility problem—it's a chest wall muscle (pectorals, etc.) and connective tissues problem—I think having good shoulder mobility definitely helped my return to normality. I was struck by how many people said to me afterward, "Wow, you healed so quickly. But you're different. You're not like me. If I had those surgeries, I would never heal that quickly." The thing is, I am *not* different. I am not special or bionic (I got cancer, after all). My body doesn't have any different healing capacity than anybody else's. I'm a mortal human just like my friends. Yes, I started with base fitness and was hyperconscious about sleeping as much as possible and increasing my protein intake to offset the muscle-wasting effects of the surgery (see page 174). But these are not heroics, just basics.

I think if there was anything different about my own recovery from surgery, it was that I made the decision to start moving immediately. That's the key to physical resilience. Within forty-eight hours of going under the knife I was riding a stationary bike (hands-free). I walked every day. My legs worked, so why not bike and walk? I also began right away to use breathing to improve my body organization. Then, as soon as I could—which the doctor told me was after six weeks—I began using very light weights and slowly moving my arms overhead. This was not because I'm obsessed with exercise or was worried about getting fat. It was because I knew from the work we do that movement increases blood flow and blood flow accelerates healing, and that not moving just allows range of motion to atrophy. With that in mind, I just kept moving, moving, and moving.

Doctors, understandably, want their patients to be cautious after surgery, but sometimes that translates into people being so timid and protective that they completely sit out the next three months, losing mobility all the while. My experience is that it's better if a doctor gives you permission to see how you feel as you go along. If I felt anything "off," I quickly stopped what I was doing. I went slowly and listened to my body.

The ideal is to never have cancer at all. But to the extent that 40 percent of us will at some point get the dreaded diagnosis—and/or have some other unexpected health-related setback during our lifetime—the more durable your body, the easier it's going to be to weather the challenge. For me, it ended up being a blip, not a catastrophic life event. I was lucky, but in recovery, I made my own luck, too.

Resolving the Shoulder-Neck Conundrum

As with a lot of predicaments the body finds itself in, breathing is key to untangling the shoulder-neck problem. If you can get into a position where you can take a big breath, it's a sign that your body is organized in such a way as to prevent muscles and joints from being inhibited, and to allow for maximum function. You might remember that we talked about "organization" in Vital Sign 2. We prefer the word "organization" to "posture," because posture is often associated with a misguided idea of military bearing that translates to being excessively taut and overly flexed and extended in some areas.

In fact, some sports and tasks in life are impossible to perform with "perfect posture." "Organized," on the other hand, means having your body be in a position where you can take a deep, full breath, and that in turn means you'll be able to tap into your innate end ranges of motion. We want to restore those end ranges—that's what all the mobilizations in this book, including the ones for the shoulders and neck, are about—but we also acknowledge that everybody has their own best positions. There is no such thing as perfect posture.

That said, we know that the rounded-upper-back C shape does not foster either good breathing or mobility. Think back to raising your arm while in a C shape versus raising your arm when your body is in a straighter silhouette. The C shape generates what we call "positional inhibition." It doesn't mean you're weak, just that the positioning of your body is prohibiting effective and forceful movement as if you *are* weak. When your body is organized into a balanced shape, you're going to have good shoulder and arm mobility, and therefore less stress on your neck. It'll make the lights come back on in the house.

There are also some other detrimental aspects of the C shape that are worth talking about. The shoulder/neck/T-spine area gets its functional integrity from three systems. One is the bony structures, like the shoulder blades and spinal column and their joints, that provide the framework of your body. Another is the muscular system, which includes not just the prime movers that the fitness world tends to focus on—the pecs, biceps, triceps, traps—but also small muscles between the vertebrae that contribute to spinal stability as well as to our awareness of where our body is in space. The third system is the connective tissue like fascia, which as it surrounds and holds muscles and organs in place helps us move. When you're curled forward in a C position for any length of time, what you end up doing is hanging on these systems (one of our Navy SEAL friends calls it "hanging on the meat"). As a result, the systems become compromised. It's like tugging on a sweater. Pull on that cardigan often and long enough, and it's going to lose its normal shape and springiness. It can still do what it's supposed to do—keep you warm—but it might not do it as well as it would if it fit properly.

When you're constantly hanging on the structural and functional systems of your upper back, those systems adapt. The C becomes the default position and, as a result, your body will eventually be unable to do all the things (other than looking at a computer) you might find interesting in life. That's why you should care. If you don't feel pain, maybe you think it doesn't matter: "As long as it doesn't hurt, I'm fine." But moving dexterously has a value all its own. You are going to be moving all your life; do it well.

Let us, though, also say this: Sometimes it's impossible for your body to be in a well-organized position for most of the day. There are jobs that don't allow it. Consider the fighter jet pilots who are cramped into a little cockpit with 10 Gs of force coming at them. Consider the receptionist whose job is to sit at a poorly designed desk for eight hours. Two sides of a not-entirely-different coin with somewhat similar problems. You can't always be in the perfect position, and that's okay. That's what the physical practice in this chapter is for. If you don't have occasion to get into healthier shapes through the natural course of the day, these targeted mobilizations for the neck and shoulders will allow you to practice them. Yes, you may have to do them more often than someone who doesn't spend freakish hours in a C shape. It's harder to turn that tanker around when it's been heading in one direction for so long. But the great news is that you can! A committed mobility practice counteracts the effects of poor positions, helping you both move your body and do so with more vigor.

And if you are experiencing pain—and neck pain in particular? When something hurts, it's always a good policy to look at what's connected to the area you want to change. (We'll talk more about the upstream/downstream approach to figuring out what's causing pain beginning on page 188.) As mentioned earlier, the neck and shoulders are a couplet, and there's good evidence to suggest that focusing on the shoulders can help resolve neck pain.

Back in 2008, Danish researchers did a study involving ninety-four women who were experiencing neck pain. (Notably, 79 percent of them worked on a keyboard for most of the day.) In the paper they published on the study, the researchers noted that a protocol of neck and shoulder strength-training exercises reduced the women's pain by 75 percent. At least the researchers called them neck and shoulder strength-training exercises—what they really were, if you read the study closely, were *shoulder* isometric exercises. What that tells us is that the shoulders are the key to a pain-free neck *and* that strengthening isometrics—not stretching the neck, which is most people's go-to remedy for neck pain—is how you make your neck feel better. One reason stiffness and lack of mobility occur in muscles is because, if you avoid movement in an area for long periods of time (i.e., never move your head side to side), the brain will put on the brakes when you try to do it. It doesn't trust that you have the range to do it. Isometrics are a great way to remind your brain that it's okay to move in certain ways, and that can help you restore native function to the area.

You can also improve shoulder mobility by increasing rotation of the arms. Most people's arms rotate forward pretty well, but rotating back (external rotation) is another story. And yet rotating the arms back slightly in their sockets is a good resting position to be in, one that fosters advantageous organization of the upper body and gives you more power in your arms. We worked on external shoulder rotation with an Olympic gold medal bobsledder, and it helped her connect more forcefully with the sled, increasing her speed. Of course, most of us won't be going ninety miles per hour down a bobsledding chute, but having more power in your arms can help you with anything, from pushing a shopping cart to, in the event you need to, pushing yourself up off the floor after a fall.

Mobilizations will help you develop better external rotation, but it's also something you can practice daily simply by reminding yourself to gently roll your arms back at the spot where your upper arms meet your shoulders. If you're carrying a laundry basket, think of trying to "snap" the basket in half. Same when you're pushing a grocery cart or stroller. This action creates external rotation in the shoulder. You know you're doing it right when the pectoral muscles in your chest lie flat and your palms face forward a bit.

While we're on the subject of external rotation, just a word to you yogis out there. If you do yoga regularly, you probably get your shoulders and neck into beneficial positions quite often. There are many poses that require you to raise your arms overhead, and downward dog is great for taking the shoulders to their end flexion range. Warrior II has you turn your head to the side. So there are lots of ways yoga can help with shoulder and neck mobility. However, there is one area where we think that yoga misinterprets how to access good shoulder mobility. Teachers often instruct students to keep their shoulder blades back and down. But the shoulder blades actually need to be able to move all over the place. A better approach is to externally rotate your arms in the sockets just as we described earlier. These are nuanced ideas, but they can make a big difference in how your body is organized and thus how well it moves.

Physical Practice: Shoulder Flexion, Upper Back, and Rotator Cuff Mobilizations

Because the way we live now truncates our movement lexicon, most of us are missing key shapes that our body is primed for. This, as we've noted throughout this chapter, is particularly true of the shoulder area. These mobilizations are designed to get the joints and muscles to move in ways that they might not otherwise on a typical day. Any tools you use—a ball, in the case of these mobilizations—simply help facilitate the movement.

While we want you to do these mobilizations as often as possible, also think of other ways you can move the shoulder and neck area, especially if you're feeling tension and stiffness. That's a signal that you need to move more. So, when you can do so safely, reach for things instead of using a stepladder. Wheel your arms around when you get out of bed in the morning to help you wake up. As you sit at your desk, roll your shoulders back like we talked about above. If you have a backup camera in your car, give it a rest sometime and turn around to look behind you when you back up (we did it before they installed those cameras; we can do it again). As you go on your walks, turn your head both ways to look at your surroundings. This will not only give your trapezius muscles a break, it'll make your walk a hundred times more pleasant.

Wall Hang

This can also be done using a counter or in the downward dog position.

Stand a few feet away from a wall. Bend at the waist and, with your back flat, place your palms flat on the wall. Keeping your head in between your arms, roll your shoulders outward (try to rotate your arms so that your elbow pits are pointing up at the sky) and "hang" on the wall. Hold for ten big breaths. Try to think about expanding your back and rib cage while you breathe.

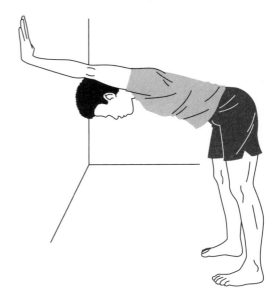

From Pilates to yoga to gymnastics and Olympic-style weightlifting, all share a common arms-overhead currency. Fortunately, this position is easy to work into your day.

T-Spine Mobilization 2

In this mobilization, you'll be using the ball to mobilize the vertebrae and soft tissue in the upper back. It also lets your arms spend time in the ever-so-important overhead position.

Lie faceup on the floor, knees bent. Place a ball on the right side at the base of your neck, just at the top of the scapula. Raise your right arm overhead and, with the thumb pointed down, drop your hand down to the floor. Keep your elbow close to your head. Raise and lower your arm at a comfortable speed, breathing as you go, ten times. Now roll back a little so the ball is farther down your back, at about the middle of your scapula. Repeat the arm raising and lowering ten times. Finally, roll back again, moving the ball to the bottom of your scapula. Repeat the arm raising and lowering ten times. Switch sides. To create a more intense mobilization, do the exercise with your butt raised off the ground in a bridge position.

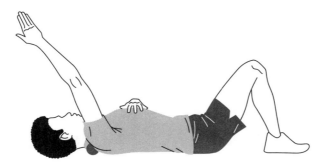

Moving the arm overhead while mobilizing the tissues of the upper back gives context to the mobilization.

Rotator Cuff Mobilization

The effect this has on shoulder rotation is stunning. We suggest following up the exercise by retaking the Shoulder Rotation Test to see how dramatic the effects are. You don't have to retake the test every time, but taking it after just doing the Rotator Cuff Mobilization your first time will show you that your efforts are not going to waste.

Lie faceup on the floor, knees bent. Place a ball under the point where your right shoulder meets your upper arm. Turn to the right side slightly so the ball sits snugly at the rotator cuff (but not under the arm). Extend your right arm out to the side, elbow bent at a 90-degree angle and your forearm perpendicular to the floor. In this position, inhale and exhale slowly as you contract, then relax the muscles sitting on the ball. Do this ten times. From there, alternate moving your forearm forward and back as far as it will go, keeping the elbow on the floor. Do this ten times. Switch sides.

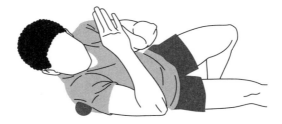

A ball in the back of the shoulder mobilizes those targeted tissues but also brings awareness to this area.

BOTTOMS UP: THE RIGHT WAY TO DO A PUSH-UP

If we handed you a big box, would you hold it with your shoulders forward and your arms out wide or would you hold it with your arms back and the box close to your body? Go ahead and simulate it both ways and see what feels right. Your arms close to your body is the most likely answer, because having your arms out is more of a strain. So why do so many people do push-ups—one of the best possible exercises for your shoulders and for building strength throughout the body—with their arms way out to the side? It's both inefficient and difficult. We think there's a better way.

Lie on the floor facedown, swing your arms out in front of you, then quickly bring them back to your sides and place them, palms down, in the position you would if you were going to raise yourself up off the floor in a hurry. That automatically puts you into the perfect push-up position. (Yogis, this is also the correct position for doing the pose chaturanga.) From there, squeeze your butt and push up off the floor into a plank position (the body straight and hovering over the floor while you are on your hands and toes). Take a breath there, then lower yourself back down until you're a few inches from the floor. Repeat. While you're doing your push-ups, imagine that your hands are flat on dinner plates and you are trying to screw those dinner plates into the ground, with your right hand "moving" clockwise and your left hand "moving" counterclockwise. This will help you attain good shoulder rotation and stability as you go.

You may need to worm and wiggle your way to reach the top of the push-up, but that's okay. We love the worm push-up! That's how we teach kids to do push-ups, and we have not met a single person who can't do one when they start at the bottom and worm their way up. Eventually you will get stronger, you'll wiggle less and less, then finally you'll be able to smoothly go up and down. If you're just beginning to do push-ups, this is a much better way to build strength than to do push-ups on your knees. Rarely does anybody ever progress to regular push-ups from the knee push-up; plus, it can cause range-of-motion problems in the shoulder. Go with the worm! Not only does this technique make for better push-ups, but it also cues us to activate our glutes, gives some extension input into our spines, and keeps some shoulder extension in our movement lexicon.

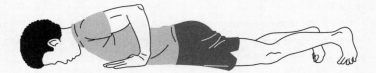

Forearms vertical allow for better and more powerful shoulder movement.

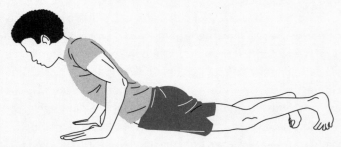

The Worm-Up is a fantastic movement that allows for great spinal hygiene, and everyone can do it!

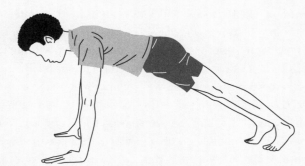

The dreaded plank. Can you breathe?

EAT LIKE YOU'RE GOING TO LIVE FOREVER

ASSESSMENT **PART 1: 800-Gram Count;**
PART 2: Protein Count

PHYSICAL PRACTICE **800-Gram Challenge; Protein Boost**

FOOD, OF COURSE, is many things to us. But putting aside for a moment its association with comfort and culture and pleasure, food at its most basic provides the building blocks of our body and the fuel that keeps it running. This is not news to you—people have been telling us we are what we eat since 1826, when the French gastronome par excellence Jean Anthelme Brillat-Savarin wrote, "Dis-moi ce que tu manges, je te dirai ce que tu es" (Tell me what you eat and I will tell you what you are). What might be news to you, though, is that what you eat relates to how you move. We couldn't credibly develop a program for improving durability and restoring mobility without addressing the food issue. Indeed, with a nod to Brillat-Savarin, you move as you eat.

Your daily nutrient intake affects all the components that allow you to move, including your muscles, tendons, ligaments, and other tissues, as well as your cartilage and bones. It also influences the level of inflammation in your body and that, too, can affect movement. And if you're not eating right, you may potentially heal more slowly from injuries or surgery, something Kelly, as a physical therapist, has run across multiple times.

On one particularly notable occasion during his first year in practice, he was treating a client who had had meniscus transplant surgery, a procedure that involves replacing the shock-absorbing cartilage around the knee. The client came in with his knee swollen and inflamed well past the time it should have been. "Why is your knee so angry?" Kelly asked, wondering what was going on. Then a lightbulb went off. "What did you have for breakfast?" he asked. "A box of cereal," the client replied. The guy had spent thousands of dollars on this costly surgery, only to eat like a teenager without a care in the world! What he thought of as "breakfast" was in reality a sugar bomb low in both protein and micronutrients. His diet wasn't providing the elements he needed to heal, and it was showing. Again, you are what you eat.

Tissues that are nourished improperly not only behave differently, but some massage therapists report they even *feel* different to the touch. A sensitive therapist can tell when a client is living on highly processed foods—they lend themselves to inflammation throughout the body, as well as other noticeable problems. Poorly hydrated and nourished tissues don't behave in the same way as hydrated and nourished tissues. Have you ever looked in the mirror the morning after a big night of pizza and beer with your friends? Your skin may not look quite as young as it did the day before! The bottom line is that, no matter what it is you're building— whether it's a human being or a house—you get better results when you use the best raw materials available.

The truth is, you can survive on just about anything, and sometimes you may need to (see Extra-Credit Assessments, page 161). But your body is kind of like the camping stove Kelly had in college. He had bought an MSR-brand stove specifically because it was a multifuel device. It ran on kerosene, white gas, even gasoline. On one camping trip, he thought, "Oh, you can burn gasoline? Let's try that." No sooner had he and his friends started to cook with the gasoline-fueled stove than black smoke began spilling out, covering their pots and clogging the fuel jet. They cleaned the jet, cooked for two minutes more, and it happened all over again. Moral of the story: Just because you *can* burn any type of fuel doesn't mean you should. You're not necessarily going to get a good outcome.

Our approach to nutrition is all about good fuel—quality nutrients. We're not fussy about the configuration of those nutrients. We are not, for example, for or against Paleo or Atkins or Mediterranean or Whole30 or Keto, or any other particular diet. We don't care if you're vegan or vegetarian or carnivore. We know people who have had success with all of the above; different things definitely work for different people. Besides the sweeping admonition "Don't base your diet on crappy, processed food," we are primarily interested in two things and two things only: protein and micronutrients. It's been our experience that when you focus on these two things, everything else—including calorie control and healthier eating habits—falls into place.

These two elements of the diet also fit into what Cate Shanahan, MD, calls the Four Pillars of World Cuisine (more generally, the Four Pillars of the Human Diet). In her book *Deep Nutrition: Why Your Genes Need Traditional Food,* Shanahan explains that just about every culture the world over eats foods that are nutritionally equivalent. They may look different—one culture's pickled turnips are another culture's kimchi; you've got pork ramen in one country, *caldo de pollo* in another—but they have commonalities, and those commonalities are no accident. As humans, we are built to thrive on the foods our ancestors so wisely sussed out, learned to properly prepare, and passed down through cultural traditions. Our DNA is waiting! Shanahan's research led her to single out these four shared elements of the optimal human diet: meat on the bone; fermented and sprouted foods; organs and other offal; fresh and unadulterated plant and animal products. While you may not subscribe to the particulars Shanahan recommends—we know organ meats, for instance, are a hard sell—you can still take away the basic tenets of her Four Pillars, which is that the body needs protein and unadulterated foods, including fruits and vegetables, our greatest source of micronutrients.

The tests and physical practices for this Vital Sign are designed to make eating simple. They don't offer a quick fix, nor were they conceived to turn you into an Instagram model with shredded abs. These are nutrition strategies for maintaining a robust, healthy body—no matter what body type nature gave you. And, again, they're designed to keep things simple. The world around us keeps manufacturing complex solutions for what should be blissfully uncomplicated. Five-hour energy drinks? Keto candy? What the . . . ? And have you walked down the supplements aisle lately? Granted, supplements can be helpful in certain circumstances, and taking a daily multivitamin can be good insurance. But nothing takes the place of real food.

At no time was this clearer to us than when we brought our younger daughter home from the hospital. She had been in the NICU for three weeks after birth, and when she was released from the hospital, the doctors sent her home with some vitamins. The vitamins tasted terrible (we weren't going to give them to her without trying them out!) and that was not something we wanted to subject our infant daughter to. And besides, by this time, she was breastfeeding heartily—in other words, in receipt of the perfect food—and it would seem she was getting all the nutrients she required.

"Why does she need these?" we asked. "Because women in San Francisco don't get any sun, so they don't make enough vitamin D," we were told. (The body manufactures vitamin D itself through sun exposure.) Oh, why didn't you say so? There was a simple solution: It was August, a notoriously foggy time in San Francisco, but we were staying up in sunny Marin County. So we protected our newborn's head and exposed her body to the sun for five minutes a day. Juliet also sat out in the sun for short periods of time so she'd produce adequate D (you only need ten to thirty minutes' exposure a few times a week). Our daughter developed into a strong, healthy baby on nothing but breastmilk (at this writing, she's thirteen years old and five foot nine). Problem solved without a complex, artificial solution.

Here's another instance where a simple solution turned out to be the better one. For a hot minute in the early 2000s, it was popular for performance athletes to use IVs to hydrate. As advertised, it was a "magical" way to get the body's fluids back up to an optimal level after workouts. Well, as it happens, when people are given fluids via IV, they still feel thirsty because their brain doesn't register the hydration. Drinking hydrates just as well *and* eliminates thirst. Once again, the complicated antidote not only takes more effort, it isn't a superior fix.

We tell you these stories not to extol the virtues of breastmilk or water bottles, but to make the case for getting back to basics. Everything you need in your diet is available at your typical, no-frills grocery store. And you can scale up from there. If you love to cook, take these simple ingredients and have at it. Same goes if you love to eat out; just keep our recommendations for protein and micronutrients in mind as you order. If you're training for a marathon, add more carbs. If you're trying to lose weight, scale back the calories. It doesn't have to be rocket science, and the payoff will be tangible.

Take the rewards of getting adequate protein. Protein figures decisively in building and maintaining muscle, and maintaining muscle, of course, figures decisively in the body's functionality. Protein also figures into sustaining other parts of the body, like all your connective tissue and the lining of your small intestine. Something we've learned when talking to people about their diets is that it's not widely known that our protein needs increase as we get older. Gradually, but early on, the body can begin to lose muscle mass. It starts when we're in our thirties and typically continues apace at a rate of about 3 to 5 percent a decade, depending on genetics, how active you are—and your protein intake. Because, while many factors figure into age-related muscle loss, one of them is a decline in the body's ability to turn dietary protein into muscle. So imagine the consequences if you're not getting enough protein to begin with.

That's why we're such big advocates for keeping the little muscle-making factories in our body well stocked. By making sure you eat enough protein throughout the years, you can help slow this inevitable part of the human condition.

Micronutrients, the other aspect of nutrition we consider high priority, also play a starring role in movement health. Micronutrients are vitamins and minerals that are essential to wellness. In plant foods, they often come accompanied by phytochemicals, compounds like flavonoids, phenolic acids, isoflavones, curcumin, isothiocyanates, and carotenoids, which have been shown to have their own health benefits. (Macronutrients are the big guns—fat, carbohydrate, and protein.) These small but mighty elements assist in the growth and development of cells, immune function, energy production, nerve conduction and muscle contraction, and hundreds of other processes that keep the body running smoothly. You can't live without them, though you can get by with minimal amounts. But who wants to just get by?

Is it good enough to just have enough vitamin C to allow you to avoid scurvy? Or do you want the amount that will help your body quickly repair tissue (including skin tissue—which is why there is often vitamin C added to skincare products)? Do you want just enough vitamin D to help you avoid rickets (the reason the U.S. began adding it to milk in the 1930s, when the bone-softening disease was rampant among poor children)? Or do you want the amount that helps protect against osteoporosis? The same goes for micronutrients. Don't settle for "just enough." If you want to have the power to fight disease, to have maximum mobility, and just to all-around *thrive*, you'll do well to get lots and lots of micronutrients.

Before we dive into the tests, let us say one more thing about our big-picture nutrition philosophy: Healthy eating is about compromise. Food should be a joy. You don't want to be the person who can't go anywhere and misses out on the bonhomie that surrounds eating because your diet is so restricted. On the other end of the spectrum, you don't want to be someone who takes no care about what you consume. The goal is to be somewhere in the middle. Find that happy place.

Assessment: Part 1: 800-Gram Count; Part 2: Protein Count

The two tests for this Vital Sign are spot checks on how well you're doing in meeting your protein and micronutrient needs. Typically, we're not ones for weighing and measuring food, but it's worth doing on occasion to see if your impressions about your diet match the reality. Because no matter if you think you're below or above the requirements or right on target, things may not always be what they seem. One of our clients who'd always considered herself a healthy eater got a rude awakening when, in preparation for knee replacement surgery, we asked her to do the micro-nutrient assessment. Turns out, the number of micronutrient-rich foods she was eating on an average day was only 100 grams, far below the 800 grams we should all be going for. She was shocked.

This is a good time to acknowledge that measuring food can be a way that some people exert control over their life. That's not what this is about, and if you have struggled with an eating disorder or found your-self using food measuring in punishingly restrictive ways at any time, just skip the tests. Perfection is not the goal here. Like all the tests in this book, the main purpose of these micronutrient food and protein counts is to bring your awareness to something you may have been ignoring or, like our knee replacement gal, simply misjudging. Just taking a look, with or without measurements, can help you see if you need to reassess and make some healthy changes.

PART 1: 800-GRAM COUNT
EC Synkowski, MS, CNS, LDN, is a Maryland-based nutrition coach who we have been consulting with for over a decade. During that time, she'd

been working on the problem of nutrition confusion: There were so many recommendations out there; how could she boil it all down to its most important essence? What EC came up with was a simple but brilliant idea. Instead of worrying about whether you're getting enough of each kind of vitamin, mineral, antioxidant, phytochemical—a minefield of recommendations that aren't easy to decode—EC created a simple, research-based benchmark that streamlines eating dictums into one easy-to-follow challenge: Eat 800 grams (by weight) of fruits and vegetables a day.

That's it. They can be fresh, cooked, frozen, or canned in water, so the options are plentiful. Because you weigh the food (though after a while you'll be so adept at eyeballing fruits and vegetables that you can dispense with the scale), you don't have to worry about serving sizes or food groups or food pyramids or any of the other confusing healthy-eating guidelines. And the beauty of EC's 800-Gram Challenge (we're calling it that since we've adapted it for this book, but it's technically the #800gChallenge®) is that it's all about *adding* to your diet. Every day there's something else we're advised to subtract from our diet, so this approach is refreshing.

Those are the basics you need to know right now in order to do the assessment. Later on in this chapter, we'll tell you more about how EC came up with that number, and some easy ways to make sure you meet it.

PREPARATION

The best way to do an accurate count of your fruit and vegetable intake is to use a kitchen scale. These are generally reasonably priced (and can come in handy when you're following a recipe that puts ingredients in weights, a more accurate way to measure than cups and spoons). However, don't sweat it if you don't have one. As a gauge, 800 grams of raw produce amounts to about 6 cups (and one cup is about the size of a fist for most produce). One caveat: Because they have a lot of volume but little weight, tally raw leafy greens, like spinach, kale, collards, and chard, as only part of what you would for something like broccoli (i.e., 5 cups spinach = 1 cup broccoli).

Choose a day to monitor that is typical of how you generally eat. The test will probably go smoother if you also do it on a day when you're not eating out or ordering in. If, however, you eat out or order in daily, then by all means figure a typical restaurant meal into your count. Just familiarize yourself with what a cup measurement looks like and eyeball any fruits and vegetables that meet the criteria on your plate.

THE TEST

Beginning with the first thing you put in your mouth in the morning and ending with the last thing you eat at night, jot down every gram of sanctioned fruit and vegetable you consume throughout the day, preferably using a scale to measure (see above). Add up the numbers and you have your score.

As you might expect, the 800-Gram Count has a few rules. For instance, Fruit Loops don't make the grade, and French fries (because they are fried, not because they're potatoes) are a nonstarter. But you probably suspected that. Here are guidelines for what else you need to know.

COUNTS	DOESN'T COUNT
Raw fruits and vegetables (even with dressings)	Dried fruits and vegetables, i.e., raisins, dates, dried peas
Cooked, frozen (without preadded sauces or seasonings), or canned (in water) fruits and vegetables	Nondairy (i.e., plant-based) milks
Fruits and vegetables incorporated into recipes such as smoothies, salsas, and soups (weigh before adding or do the math by looking at the recipe and dividing the amount of produce by the number of servings)	Juice
Tofu	Jellies and jams
Beans	Fried vegetables like French fries and tempura (the unhealthiness of the frying cancels out the healthiness of the veggies)

COUNTS	DOESN'T COUNT
Tomato sauce without added oil or sugar	Grains
Fruits and vegetables often left off other nutrition lists: potatoes, corn, (non-dried) edamame, peas, avocados	All types of flours (including almond and chickpea)
Pickles and fermented vegetables like kimchi	Pastas made from vegetables
Olives	Nuts and seeds
Fruit compotes (like applesauce) made without sugar	Popcorn

WHAT YOUR RESULTS MEAN

Your score is the number of grams you eat per day.

There's little room for nuance here. You're either eating 800 grams of fruits and vegetables or you're not. If you're getting 800 or more grams a day, you're golden. You've hit the mark and, as long as you are not also eating tons of processed foods to nullify the goodness of the produce, just keep doing what you're doing. If you're not hitting 800 grams, ramp it up until you are. We'll give you some ideas on how to do it later in this chapter.

WHEN SHOULD YOU RETEST?

Measure your grams every day until you feel that you have a comfortable knowledge of what constitutes 800 grams.

PART 2: PROTEIN COUNT

Just about everyone gets some protein in their diet, but in our estimation many people are still coming up short. We should say up front that there are differing ideas about what constitutes the proper amount of protein per day. Our recommendation—between 0.7 and 1 gram of protein per pound of body weight—falls somewhere in between the U.S. Department of Agriculture's conservative daily allowance (about 0.4 grams per 1 pound of body weight) and the guy at your gym encouraging you to, like him, knock back protein shakes all day. That is, our recommendation is higher than guidelines for the general public but is safe, well within reason, and based on studies that indicate the USDA guidelines may be behind the times. (See page 169 for more on our protein rec.)

Protein, of course, is the macronutrient contained in high amounts in red meat, poultry, and seafood and, in lesser quantities, dairy products. Grains, particularly whole grains, also contain some protein, as do nuts, seeds, beans, legumes (like lentils, peanuts, soybeans, peas), and some vegetables. In this assessment, we ask you to add up grams of protein from all sources. If you use protein powder (see Protein Powder—Thumbs Up or Down?, page 175), throw those grams in there, too.

PREPARATION

You'll need a system for measuring protein and a way (calculator, pencil and paper) of adding up the grams from disparate foods. Gauging how much protein you eat in a day requires a little more legwork than counting fruit and vegetable grams. Although you can weigh some of your pure protein sources—it's easy, for instance, to slap a chicken thigh or flank steak on your kitchen scale and add the number to your tally, since almost all the weight in these foods is protein—other sources of protein may require some research. For instance, your breakfast cereal may contain protein, so you'll need to check the nutrition facts on the side of the box to get the amount. Even vegetables can contain some protein (a cup of broccoli has 2 grams), and there are also mixed dishes to consider. How much protein is in your bean and cheese burrito? (Beans 7 grams + cheese 7 grams + tortilla 1 gram = 15 grams.) Besides food labels, the USDA's FoodData Central website's search engine (fdc.nal.usda.gov) can help you with your calculations, as can the various websites (like myfooddata.com) and apps (such as MyFitnessPal) that provide nutrient data.

You can also use some visual cues to help you. A serving of fish, chicken, or meat that's the size of your palm is approximately 3 ounces, or 23 grams. A half cup of beans and legumes is about the size of your fist, and beans and lentils have between 7.5 and 8.5 grams of protein per half cup.

As with the earlier test, choose a day to monitor that is typical of how you generally eat, whether that involves restaurants or meals prepared at home or some combination of the two. Be honest with yourself and opt for a day that reflects your real life.

THE TEST

Beginning with the first thing you put in your mouth in the morning and ending with the last thing you eat at night, jot down every gram of protein you consume throughout the day. This includes all forms of protein, vegetarian or nonvegetarian, and also includes protein supplements, if you use them. Add up the numbers and you have your score.

WHAT YOUR RESULTS MEAN

Base your scoring on this formula: Between 0.7 and 1 gram of protein per pound of body weight. If you don't move much during the day, it's okay to hit the lower end of the range. If you exercise moderately (i.e., hike or pedal a Peloton for thirty minutes or the equivalent a few times a week), you should be leaning into the middle. And if you're an athlete, are prepping for or recovering from surgery, or are over sixty, you want to be striving for the top end of the range.

As with the 800-Gram Count, the scoring here is black-and-white. You're either reaching your optimal number of grams per day or not, and your goal should be to hit the mark. This is not to discount getting close or improving as you go. However, we urge you to aim high and work to meet your target protein count.

WHEN SHOULD YOU RETEST?

Measure your protein grams every day until you feel that you have a comfortable knowledge of what constitutes your daily requirement.

EXTRA-CREDIT ASSESSMENTS: FRAPPUCCINO TEST; 24-HOUR FAST

As we've stated often and in various ways, one of the aims of this book is to help you get to know yourself better from a physiological standpoint. Your mission now, should you choose to accept it (these are totally optional tests), is to get a window into something called your "metabolic flexibility."

Metabolic flexibility is best described as the body's ability to adapt fuel utilization to changes in fuel availability. What that means in real-life terms is if you have strong metabolic flexibility, you should be able to wake up in the morning, eat nothing, and go do your workout or go to work without bonking (which means becoming exhausted, usually because of poor fueling). You should also be able to handle foods that are what we might call over-the-top in fat and calories (like a Frappuccino) without feeling sick to your stomach or having diarrhea.

This is something many great athletes can attest to. As legendary big-wave surfer Laird Hamilton likes to point out, if the only food available to you is a Big Mac and your digestive system has become so precious that you can't handle it, you're going to be in trouble, because the perfect foods are not always available, especially when you're on the road. If you're working with a group, as Laird does when using Jet Skis for tow-in surfing, you can be a liability if you bonk. Ultramarathoner Dean Karnazes famously ordered a pizza to be delivered to him during a 200-mile race. Although he has since changed his ways—*Sports Illustrated* reported that his fridge looked like a hijacked Whole Foods warehouse and Karnazes himself has said he recovers better if he doesn't eat a lot of sugar—his legendary pizza refuel points up the benefits of metabolic flexibility. It's not that these athletes or we advocate eating these types of foods regularly—to the contrary. Choose the best possible fuel whenever possible. But we are also built to be omnivores and to be able, when necessary, to eat what's available. The body is not as sensitive as you might think.

Put another way, we evolved to thrive under erratic circumstances. In prehistoric times, some days there was an animal to eat, some days only plants, some days little to nothing at all. Our bodies had to be flexible, and because they were, they were able to produce more energy, have fewer food cravings, and still operate optimally no matter what kind of fuel they were given. Even if humans' circumstances have changed, these aspects of metabolic flexibility are still worth working toward, particularly when you consider that metabolic *in*flexibility is a characteristic of diabetes.

When you have metabolic flexibility, you'll also be less likely to feel the need to snack all the time or to refuel while doing something relatively simple, like a two-hour hike, because your blood sugar stays on an even keel. Endurance athletes, to be sure, need to plan their nutrition well, and that usually includes refueling during a long workout, but even some of them are knocking back GU and other kinds of replenishers all too often. In short, with metabolic flexibility you don't have to take in as many calories, and you'll likely find it easier to control your body weight.

How is metabolic flexibility achieved? The physical practices in this chapter—getting your micronutrient count up by eating 800 grams of fruits and vegetables per day and monitoring your protein intake—promote metabolic flexibility by packing your primary diet with healthy whole foods, leaving less room for the high-sugar, highly processed foods that send your blood sugar on an unhealthy roller-coaster ride. Eating regular meals, rather than eating meals and snacking all day long and/or propping yourself up with afternoon caffeine, also fosters metabolic flexibility.

Ready to see how you do? Here are the two assessments.

1. Frappuccino Test

This test is related to a test that doctors often give patients called the "glucose challenge test." The patients consume a sugary liquid, which causes their level of blood glucose (another name for blood sugar) to rise. This rise signals the pancreas to send the hormone insulin to work, its job being to clear glucose from the blood and help it enter the muscles and other parts of the body where it's used for energy. This lowers the blood glucose level, which is exactly what you want to happen, because having a high level for extended periods of time causes damage to the blood vessels and increases the risk of diabetes and other diseases. When blood glucose does stay high, it's usually a sign of insulin resistance, a condition where the cells fail to respond to insulin's delivery of glucose. The pancreas makes more insulin to cover the lapse, but over time its efforts can become futile and insulin resistance can turn into full-blown type 2 diabetes.

The Frappuccino Test is not a medical test, but rather just a way to gauge whether you can sugar up without feeling ill or experiencing any drastic highs and lows. The test is not going to tell you whether or not you have insulin resistance per se. But because diabetes is just crushing the planet—especially in the U.S., where it affects over 10 percent of the population—we think the test can help raise your awareness about insulin resistance and even help you see if you have any of the symptoms. After you consume the drink, you shouldn't find it hard to focus or feel nervous or moody (if you're sensitive to caffeine, order a kid's Frappuccino, which doesn't have coffee)—those are signs that sugar may not be clearing from your blood. You can get a more accurate reading by using a blood sugar monitor, available at any drugstore. In any case, if you do suspect that you are insulin resistant, check in with your healthcare provider.

PREPARATION
We chose the Starbucks Frappuccino for this test, but any similar sugar bomb can work. A regular 16-ounce Frappuccino has 45 grams of sugar; if you want to go all out, the 24-ounce has 59 (specialty flavors can have even more). Run the test on an empty stomach, at least four hours out from your last meal, and prepare not to eat again for another four hours.

THE TEST
Simply drink up and record how you feel during the next four hours.

WHAT YOUR RESULTS MEAN

Ask yourself this question: How did you feel after the Frappuccino? If you felt irritable, nauseous, jittery, or spacey, or you had diarrhea, this is an indication that you're metabolically inflexible. If you were able to get on with the business of your day without incident, you are most likely metabolically flexible. There's one red herring here. If you already live on Frappuccinos and the like, you may not experience any problems. The body does adapt, although not always the way you want it to. Does that mean you've got a healthy lifestyle going on? No. And are you sure you're not feeling any repercussions? It may be that eating junk really does make you feel terrible; you've just learned to live with it. Now's the time to reassess.

Hopefully, this small experiment has given you some insight into how your body copes with food. Whether you had problems with the Frappuccino or not, make sure you're following the 800-gram fruit and vegetable challenge and meeting your protein needs. That's going to ensure that you stay metabolically flexible or achieve it over time. If the Frappuccino pushed the envelope of your tolerance, take the test again after two weeks of following the Vital Sign 6 physical practice; things are likely to improve.

2. 24-Hour Fast

Throughout human history people have always done some form of voluntary fasting, whether it be out of religious tradition (Ramadan, Yom Kippur), as part of a spiritual discipline (some Hindus fast one day a week), or for weight loss (intermittent fasting—see page 185). Bearing in mind that, in a world where food insecurity has not abated, it is a privilege to fast for health-related self-discovery, we're asking you to try it out for twenty-four hours with an explicit goal in mind: to evaluate your relationship with food.

Not eating for a big chunk of time was once very much a part of the human experience; it's in our DNA, so we should all be tough enough to handle it. If you're not, don't feel bad about it. In our culture, we've gotten to the point where not only have we become very precious about food, restricting everything from gluten to dairy, on top of that we can't go five hours without eating. As Michael Easter points out in his book *The Comfort Crisis: Embrace Discomfort to Reclaim Your Wild, Happy, Healthy Self*, most people rarely leave their comfort zone of 72 degrees Fahrenheit, carry anything heavy, risk boredom, contemplate death—or allow their stomachs to rumble a bit with hunger. We've lost this ability to be flexible as humans. There's a big push behind the idea that we should eat three meals and two snacks a day, or even eat every three hours to "rev up our metabolism." We're bombarded with food images and actual food—the candy on a coworker's desk, the eye-catching snacks at the gas station, the pastries piled high next to the coffee shop cash register. Is it any wonder that people often eat mindlessly, whether hungry or not?

And it's a way of life many are passing down to their kids. There's a mistaken notion, too, that exercise requires constant fueling. Look, if your personal experience is that you bonk without food, we don't want to tell you not to eat. But if you're just practicing preventive consumption, you should give this extra food intake a pass and see what happens. Most people don't need it. Even the most highly trained athletes in the world go easy on food on game day, eating a slice of orange or having a sip of juice during halftime. (More on this in Coda: Thoughts on Weight Control, Intermittent Fasting, and Snacking, page 182.)

The 24-Hour Fast is not designed to be a test of willpower but rather a test of whether you're in possession of metabolic flexibility and whether, psychologically (because we know you can handle it physiologically, even if it feels bad), you can do without food for a day (drinking noncaloric beverages is okay). We're not necessarily telling you to jump on the intermittent fasting bandwagon (see page 185), but there are good reasons to go for blocks of time without eating. For instance, one thing you want your body to do is to tap into stored fat, but it doesn't need to if you're constantly throwing snacks, especially high-carb snacks, down the pipe.

Being able to handle gap times in eating is a tool that can also help you when the food pickings are not great. Say you're at the airport, have a five-hour flight ahead, and there's nothing nutritious in the offerings by your gate. You should be able to just get on the flight and skip the pretzels or the greasy chicken sandwich and be fine.

Taking a break from your regular eating rituals also lets you honestly assess hunger versus ritual. Are you really hungry or is your 3 p.m. raid on the vending machines just a way to battle midafternoon boredom or burnout? Maybe you really are hungry, but give yourself a chance to find out, instead of eating according to a metronome's beat. Take these twenty-four hours to gather some insight.

PREPARATION
Choose a day when you won't be having any social engagements that involve food or any physically or psychologically demanding projects.

THE TEST
Have a normal meal the night before your fast, then plan to have your next meal at about the same time the following day (i.e., 6 p.m. Friday, 6 p.m. Saturday). By all means have your morning coffee (no milk of any kind, or sugar) and drink as many noncaloric beverages (though none with artificial sweeteners) throughout the day as you like. Record how you feel during the day.

WHAT YOUR RESULTS MEAN
Once again, there's no point system, but your reaction to a day without eating will give you some clues to your metabolic flexibility. If in the absence of food you develop crazy cravings and find your energy level crashing big time, it's a sign of metabolic inflexibility. If you felt slightly

uncomfortable, maybe a little spacey, but didn't suffer any big swings, you have a more adaptable system.

If the fast didn't go well, consider that you need to reassess how often you're eating and what types of foods you're consuming. Granted, everyone's body is different—you could be doing everything right and still struggle with a one-day fast. This is all about taking some time to observe yourself, see what's going right, what's going wrong, and what you might want to do differently.

The Fruit and Vegetable Advantage

You've undoubtedly been urged many times to pile your plate high with produce. It's in the cultural zeitgeist; every kid learns about it in school. Nonetheless, we'd be remiss if we didn't remind you of some of the most salient reasons you should eat plenty of fruits and vegetables. So let's recap.

At a minimum, fruits and vegetables contain the vitamins and minerals that keep all systems in the body humming along. They help build DNA and hormones, allow us to turn food and oxygen into energy, assist in maintaining bone and clotting blood, keep our fluids balanced . . . the list is long. Every time you bite into a peach or slurp up a forkful of spinach, you are also ingesting properties that keep you from contracting deficiency-related diseases. Who can forget the fifth-grade lessons about explorers on produce-parched ships who suffered from the horrible effects of scurvy? It wouldn't have happened if they'd had access to vitamin C–rich fruits and veggies. But the protection of micronutrients goes beyond basic maintenance and deficiency-related ills.

EC Synkowski based the 800-Gram Challenge on a 2017 study published in the *International Journal of Epidemiology*. The researchers analyzed ninety-five studies and concluded that eating 800 grams of fruits and vegetables a day was associated with a lower risk of cardiovascular disease, some cancers, and, in fact, all causes of death. In particular, apples, pears, citrus fruits, green leafy vegetables, salads, and cruciferous vegetables (like broccoli and cauliflower) lowered cardiovascular disease and incidence of death; green and yellow vegetables and cruciferous vegetables were associated with lowering cancer risk. Research has long suggested that produce has a protective effect, not just against heart disease and cancer but also other maladies like diabetes and stroke. One of the values of this study is that it gives us something to aim for: 800 grams. Those in the nutrition world disagree about a lot of the particulars, but it's safe to say that no one opposes the idea of a diet with 800 grams of fruits and vegetables.

It turns out, too, that while protein may be the nutrient we most associate with strength and power, fruits and vegetables may also play an important role in maintaining muscle. For instance, a 2015 Japanese study found that eating soy products and green and yellow vegetables was associated with less age-related decline in muscle strength. Other studies have also shown that older adults with high fruit and vegetable intakes are at a lower risk of frailty. And the body-bolstering effects of fruits and vegetables don't just belong to the over-seventy set.

The Study of Women's Health Across the Nation, known as the SWAN study, is a project jointly sponsored by the National Institute on Aging, the National Institute of Nursing Research, the National Institutes of Health, and other groups. Specifically designed to look at women's health during their middle years, the ongoing collection of studies began in 1994 and includes women of many different ethnicities who live in varying parts of the country. In one particular investigation, SWAN researchers looked at the impact of diet on functionality, defined as being able to do things like walk, climb, lift, and carry. Their subjects were 2,160 women ages forty-two to fifty-two. The researchers assessed the women's food intake, then checked in on them four years later to see how they were doing. The results showed that the lower their fruit, vegetable, and fiber intake, the less functionality the women had only a short time down the line. In fact, someone who ate one daily serving of vegetables was 50 percent more likely to have physical limitations than someone who ate just 2.4 servings. The association was that strong.

This isn't to suggest that eating produce will suddenly give you super-powers, but it is part and parcel of an overall regimen for building and maintaining a body that moves well. And speaking of moving well, we really haven't talked about fiber yet. You may have noticed that one of the elements that predicted functionality in that SWAN study was fiber. Fiber is the cellulose, lignin, and pectin parts of fruits and vegetables (and whole grains) that are impervious to digestive enzymes and do things like help move waste out of the body, keep blood sugar levels stable, and absorb heart-imperiling cholesterol. Because it takes up a lot of space, fiber also helps keep you full, potentially lowering your calorie intake (fiber itself doesn't have any calories).

That's another thing we like about EC's 800-Gram Challenge. By eating more fruits, vegetables, and fiber, you're going to feel fuller, you're going to snack less (if at all—we rarely feel the need to), and you're going to improve the overall quality of your diet. And you just feel like you're getting so much food! You could eat a whole pound of cherries (about 450 grams) and only have consumed 225 calories. You're not going to be calling Uber Eats after that.

Protein for All

Recently someone on Instagram posted the idea that a study indicating a vegetarian diet is more cardioprotective than a nonvegetarian diet should be taken with a grain of salt (yes, the pun was intended). Let's just say the ensuing comments got emotional, with one person finally asking, "U made this just to trigger ppl right?"

If you want to step on a land mine, all you have to do is venture into the nutrition arena, where no topic is quite as fraught as protein: how much, what kinds, and when to eat it. As for the aforementioned vegetarian/nonvegetarian argument, we have no horse in that race. To eat meat or not is a personal choice, one many people make regardless of whether one is healthier than the other. And we respect that. We do, however, want to note that it's harder to meet your protein requirements with only vegetarian sources (though it can be done), and one thing we *do* believe in is meeting your protein requirements. You don't have to be heroic, never missing a gram, but being consistent is a worthy goal.

Personally, we include lean animal foods among our protein sources and there are a couple of reasons why. While you can always find studies with results that argue against the inclusion of meat in a healthy diet, there are also some convincing studies that show the opposite is true, particularly as you grow older. In Italy, researchers followed over a thousand adults, with an average age of seventy-five, for twenty years and found that eating animal protein was associated with living longer. In fact, the study, published in 2022, indicated that animal protein was *inversely* related with all causes of death, including cardiovascular disease.

Dropping for a moment the subject of protein sources, there's something that everyone agrees on: Protein is a critical macronutrient. Protein's power comes from the chains of amino acids that make up its base. Amino acids are twenty different types of molecules that link together in various combinations to create different types of protein. We are able to make some amino acids ourselves, but we must obtain others from food. The ones we get from food are called "essential amino acids" (EAAs). When we eat protein foods, the body breaks them down, freeing the EAAs, which in combination with the amino acids we make ourselves work to keep us alive and thriving. Among their most important jobs, amino acids:

- are used to produce enzymes, which enable chemical reactions in the body
- contribute to the creation of antibodies

- are an essential ingredient in the hormones that keep the body running
- facilitate the expression of DNA
- build structural components of cells and tissues, including muscle
- help muscles contract and relax

Given this list, it's readily apparent that skimping on protein can adversely affect your body in myriad ways. But since our emphasis is mobility, let's elaborate on how protein plays a role in movement. Our society is single-minded about body composition, which is to say that the focus is on losing fat. It would be so much better for our health if more of us focused less on losing fat and more on gaining muscle. And this is not only because muscle is calorie hungry—the more muscle you have, the more fat you burn—or the fact that when you lose weight on a diet, you lose both fat *and* muscle. Rather, it's primarily because muscle is so protective, and muscle loss—the medical term is "sarcopenia"—can be so debilitating. The body's process of building muscle begins to falter when we're in our thirties. The slowdown is marked by a loss of muscle mass and strength and a decrease in the quality of muscle. As we grow older, sarcopenia accelerates and becomes associated with decreased mobility and an increased risk of injury. Ultimately, people who have suffered a great deal of muscle loss lose their independence, too.

The best way to stave off muscle loss is by actively building muscle through resistance training with weights or loading by rucking. Running, swimming, cycling, walking, yoga, and other types of exercise can all help you gain and preserve some muscle, but nowhere near as effectively as resistance training. (That's why top athletes typically strength train no matter what their sport.) But whether you're disposed or not to pick up weights, you can at least make headway in keeping the muscle you have by getting sufficient dietary protein. Muscle building through exercise is a bonus; muscle maintenance through diet is base camp, something everyone can and should do. You don't have to leave muscle loss to fate, to consign it to the things written on the winds of change. You can control it!

While we talk a lot about muscle, consider, too, that ligaments, tendons, connective tissue, cartilage—other body parts that are integral to how well you can move—are also all built out of protein. Which means that the slowdown of the protein synthesis process can play out in many different ways. If, for instance, you don't want your feet to hurt, you need to make sure you have the building blocks of the connective tissue so instrumental in foot health. Your skin and the collagen that keeps it plumped up also depend on protein—so, if nothing else, let vanity drive you to meet your protein needs. With conscious eating you'll get a durable body that goes the distance *and* look your best.

Something else to consider when contemplating the role you want protein to play in your diet: satiety. Among the three macronutrients—carbohydrates, fat, and protein—protein is the one that appeases your appetite best and with the fewest calories. The science behind this is well established. Protein stimulates the release of hormones that tell you to stop eating while also decreasing the hormones that tell you to head to the refrigerator. In other words, it makes you end your meal sooner and staves off hunger for your next meal. Good news for vegetarians and vegans in this area, too. Some research suggests that nonmeat sources of protein are equally as satiating as meat proteins.

The Burning Question: How Much Protein Is Best?

Given everything we are trying to help you achieve with this book—easier movement, less musculoskeletal pain, overall good health—our recommendation for optimal protein intake is, just to remind you, 0.7 to 1 gram per pound of body weight. You may have heard lower recommendations: Major health organizations like the USDA tend to err on the side of caution and propose fewer grams (again, 0.4 grams per 1 pound of body weight). And you may have heard higher: Some athletes ramp up their protein to double the amount of our numbers. Our recommendation falls squarely in the middle. Looking at the research ourselves, asking nutrition experts for advice, and taking into consideration what's worked best for our clients, we feel that it's an optimal range, effective—and safe. An overload of protein (and just what exactly constitutes an overload has been poorly defined) stresses the kidneys, but the range we suggest is well within the safety zone.

So why a range versus one across-the-board number? Although there may be disagreement about the number of protein grams per day we should consume, there is broader consensus on the fact that a few groups of people need more protein than others. Among those groups are seniors, who need extra protein to help them maintain muscle. If you're over sixty, we recommend hitting the higher end of our protein range (1 gram per pound).

The principles behind this recommendation are important for everyone to understand, so if you're not a senior, don't skip ahead—this will be news you can use in the future, and it may even apply to you right now. As noted earlier, the human body begins to lose muscle mass after age thirty. The loss can become particularly acute beginning at age sixty-five; however, if you're inactive, you can potentially be looking at a lot of muscle loss as young as age fifty. You may even notice some related changes earlier. A woman in her forties came to us with a not uncommon problem: "I used to get strong and toned really easily," she told us. "But now, after a lapse, I recently started exercising again, and it isn't working anymore."

Maintaining muscle mass, strength, and power as we get past our middle years is not easy, but it's even more of an uphill battle if we don't have the right building blocks. With age, our bodies become less sensitive to the hormones that stimulate muscle synthesis. That means we've got to throw more raw materials into the machine if we want to crank out the same end product. Our recommendation to the woman frustrated by the lack of results from her hard work at the gym was that she increase her protein intake, which on examination proved to be below our baseline rec. After a few weeks, everything changed. She got the results she was looking for and without having to exercise any harder or more often than she already was.

Another time in life when protein needs increase is before and after undergoing surgery. Not only does the body use protein to produce collagen, which is essential for scar formation, protein's amino acids also help repair tissues touched by the doctor's scalpel and, through the formation of antibodies, assist in the prevention of post-operative infections. It's common practice for doctors to recommend that patients raise their protein intake pre- and post-surgery to help with wound healing. If you have surgery in your future, you, too, should go for the higher end of the range, beginning a few weeks before your operation date.

The last group of people who need to think about consuming in the higher range of protein is athletes and heavy-duty exercisers. If you're a moderate exerciser—say you take hikes, spend thirty minutes mountain biking, or go to yoga class a few times a week—you'll do well with the midrange amount of protein (0.8 to 0.9 grams per pound). But if you're a triathlete or work out hard for over an hour every day, consider the end range. The body constantly breaks down old muscle cells and rebuilds them with new proteins. Strenuous exercise, because it damages muscle tissue, amplifies this process in a good way—it's the breakdown of muscle that enables the body to adapt, getting stronger and better at handling the stress of activity. But the added repairs also increase the need for amino acids and thus the demand for more dietary protein.

Exercisers also need to be aware of something called the "anabolic window." Some research suggests that consuming protein within thirty minutes of ending a workout will help accelerate muscle repair. We're proponents of getting 20 to 30 grams of protein immediately after exercise, all the better if you either get it in the form of a protein drink or accompany your protein source with at least 8 ounces of water. Protein synthesis works fastest and most effectively when the muscles are hydrated.

PROTEIN POWDER—THUMBS UP OR DOWN?

One of the rules we live by is "real food first." No supplement can ever take the place of an actual food with all its complex nutrients, not to mention gustatory pleasures. But when it's a choice between not hitting our protein marks because of time constraints, a dearth of groceries in the house, or finding ourselves in a place where the real thing is not available, we are gung-ho about protein powder. This is especially true now that there are so many high-quality versions on the market, with ingredients like collagen and whey from grass-fed cows.

Supplementing with protein powder is really a busy person's strategy. On those mornings when there's not an egg to be found in the refrigerator or when our teenage daughters are set to rush out the door without eating, shakes bolstered with protein powder (or premade protein shakes) are a lifesaver. Later in the day, our family's protein will come from lean meats and some vegetarian sources, but, in the meantime, we don't have to worry about meeting our amino acid needs or get tempted to fill in the blanks with a stop at the local donut shop.

Protein powders are made with varying ingredients. Some are based on whey (a milk derivative), some with casein (another milk derivative), some with egg protein, and others with vegetarian sources of protein. This array of choices makes supplementing an option for everyone, even if you're vegetarian or vegan or have allergies. This is notable since it can be difficult to meet the 0.7 to 1 gram per pound recommendation for protein if you don't eat any animal products or even if you eat just a few. There's a lot of arguing and nitpicking over whether plant-based protein powders are as nutritious as whey-based powders, made from milk protein. And it's true, most plant-based powders don't offer the whole array of essential amino acids needed to chain together to make a complete protein (there are nine EAAs we need to get from food; the body makes the other eleven itself). But the fact is, you don't need to get all your essential amino acids from one meal—you can make up the difference by eating other protein-rich foods later.

And research suggests that some plant-based proteins—also an important option for people with lactose intolerance or dairy allergies— may actually do the job pretty well. Results have been mixed in studies looking at whether, in tandem with strength training, soy-based protein powders measure up to whey-based powders in terms of boosting muscle mass, but two studies found that pea-based protein is just as effective as whey-based protein in promoting muscle strength and thickness.

The research is still in its infancy, so if you're using plant-based protein powder, you might want to err on the side of caution by either using more of it or mixing different types. Researchers at Maastricht University in the Netherlands compared the EAAs in whey, casein, soy, and pea protein powders and found that they have, respectively, 43, 34, 27, and 30 percent of the EAAs. The EAAs in each, however, differ, so if you want to go the extra mile (and like reading labels), it can be worth your while to mix and match different powders. But frankly, don't worry about it too much, because you will still benefit. We worked with a Canadian hockey team where many of the players were lactose intolerant, so we had them use a vegetarian protein powder. They did fine and it was a lot better than having them become sick from the dairy-based powder.

Now, what to do with protein powders? The most obvious way to use one is in a smoothie or shake. But you can also stir protein powder into hot cereal and soups, mix a scoopful into pancake or muffin batter, or sprinkle it into yogurt or a bowl of cold cereal. Really, the sky's the limit—you'll just need to experiment to see how you like the taste (if you notice it at all). You can also purchase ready-made protein shakes, which is the remedy we recommended for one harried executive we were working with. He was traveling constantly, had little time for eating, and was losing weight and muscle mass as a result. Was it the best food in the world? No. But it was better than going hungry or resorting to grab-and-go junk food. It served a short-term purpose.

Physical Practice: 800-Gram Challenge and Protein Boost

Just to reiterate, these physical practices are all about *expanding* your food choices, not restricting them. If that idea strikes fear in a heart that's used to being encouraged to do the opposite, particularly if you've struggled with your weight, you can relax. You'll be adding foods that help you stave off hunger. For many, that ends up in weight loss. Here are the particulars.

800-GRAM CHALLENGE

So, what does 800 grams of fruits and vegetables look like? A lot of food (but not a lot of calories). Best-case scenario, it will also look like a beautiful mosaic—different-colored plants have different nutrients, so you get the most out of your fruits and vegetables if you mix it up. The easiest way to hit 800 grams is to include fruits and vegetables at every meal and snack. Remember, too, that beans, tomato sauce, and things like pickles and kimchi count (refresh your memory with the chart on page 157). To perhaps state the obvious, salads and vegetable soups, especially ones with an array of veggies, are a great way to pack a lot of produce in one meal. In our household, we also use the three-vegetable rule at dinner: No matter what it is we're dishing up that night, it must include three vegetables. It really helps us stay on target.

A few other things that have helped us are suggestions from Stan Efferding. Stan, who himself has been named the world's strongest body-builder, is an expert in sports nutrition and has kept many an athlete on a healthy-eating path. But you don't have to be an athlete to benefit from two particular tenets of Stan's program.

The first one: Plan ahead. Make sure you have nutritious food available by bringing it along. That may mean stashing one, maybe even a few containers in your bag so that you don't end up at the snack bar at the park while watching your kid's soccer game. If you know the only place on your

1 cup blueberries (148 g)
2 carrots, cut into sticks (144 g)
1 cup chickpeas (160 g)
1½ cups broccoli (124 g)
2 cups romaine lettuce (94 g)
1½ cup cantaloupe (160 g)

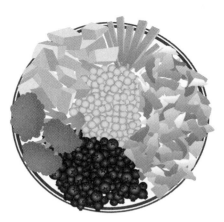

1 medium apple (182 g)
1 cup mango chunks (165 g)
1 cup sliced red pepper (92 g)
3 cups raw spinach (90 g)
1 cup sliced cucumber (119 g)
1 sweet potato (130 g)
½ cup mushroom slices (35 g)

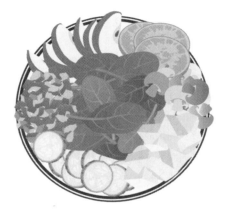

2 small tangerines (76 g)
1 cup cauliflower rice (200 g)
1 cup cherry tomatoes (149 g)
1 cup zucchini spirals (85 g)
1 cup cooked kale (130 g)
1 cup black beans (172 g)

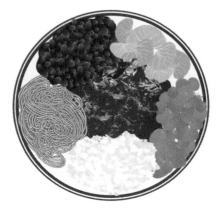

five-hour road trip is a fast-food joint known for its greasy tacos, pack a container. If you hit the gym first thing in the morning, then go straight to work, you can skip the pastry cart because *you packed your breakfast.* Making several meals at a time—as long as you're making one, why not make three?—and packing up a couple of them for later is a great way to ensure that you are never left at the mercy of unhealthy options.

The second guideline of Stan's that we also think is important is to eat foods that you can easily digest. If you're consuming foods that are causing you indigestion, gas, and bloating, cross them off your list—not only because they're making you miserable (reason enough), but because if it gets to the point where you're taking antacids, there's a good chance the medication will interfere with the breakdown of protein and the absorption of certain nutrients, like calcium, magnesium, and iron. When it comes to vegetables, Stan notes that the easiest to digest are spinach, squash, carrots, cucumbers, potatoes (which have three times the potassium of bananas), and bell peppers.

If, however, you have no digestion problems, the sky's the limit when it comes to fruit and vegetables. In that vein, see the facing page for a few examples of what constitutes 800 grams of produce.

PROTEIN BOOST

We've talked a great deal about the why of protein; now let's talk about the what—as in, "What should I eat?" We are not endorsing any particular sources here, but obviously it will be easier to meet your daily requirement if you choose foods naturally high in protein, which puts animal protein at the top of the list. Animal proteins not only have the most protein per serving, they also are "complete"—they contain all nine of the essential amino acids the body needs for muscle synthesis and other functions. If you don't eat animal protein, you still have plenty of options (check out some of the most protein-packed ones in the charts below). Just be aware that vegetarian/vegan sources aren't complete; however, because different foods have different amino acids, you will most likely get them all through the course of the day. This is where variety can be your friend: The more diverse your diet, the greater diversity of nutrients it will provide.

Keep in mind that by increasing your protein intake you're doing something positive for your health, so don't muck it up by choosing protein sources so fatty or processed that you're effectively canceling out the benefits. (The protein in that double-decker cheeseburger with bacon may help you maintain muscle, but come on! Your heart!) Also be careful about nullifying the calorie-saving benefits of protein by overdoing it with healthy but high-calorie protein sources. Nuts and seeds, for instance. Nutritious as they are, because of their naturally high oil content (raw nuts and seeds included), we count them as fats. This isn't to say you should never eat them (especially if you don't eat animal foods, they can be a good vegetarian source of protein); however, be real about how much you're eating. Do you know how many calories are in a teaspoon of peanut butter? About 31. No big deal, *except nobody ever eats a teaspoon of peanut butter.* More like four tablespoons (376 calories). We're not fatphobic—fat helps the body absorb nutrients, so please keep the skin on your chicken breast, go for the dark meat, and so on. Just do everything within reason.

Remember, too, that protein has that great satiating effect, so use it to your advantage to keep your calories in check. When our oldest daughter was a newborn, we were invited to attend a holiday party in the apartment upstairs from Juliet's mother. In the elevator on the way up to the festivities, Juliet turned to Kelly and was startled by the way he looked. "What's wrong with your cheeks?" They were stuffed with pork. Scrambling to get out of the house on time and with an infant in one hand, Kelly had tried to gobble down some food before the party. The party, of course, would have food—which was just what he was hoping to avoid. What likely awaited was the dreaded cheese plate (perfectly delicious, perhaps, but pretty much an explosion of cholesterol and calories). By downing some appetite-quenching protein pre-party, he knew it would give him the will to resist the cheese extravaganza. It's a strategy we've both used ever since (though now Kelly manages to finish chewing before leaving the house).

As you go about proteining up your diet, try to spread out your protein sources throughout the day. Some research suggests that the body builds more muscle if protein is consumed at intervals. It's not conclusive, but it makes sense even just on a practical level. The more committed you are to having protein at every meal, the more likely you'll hit your target.

Here's everything you need to know going forward.

DAILY PROTEIN REQUIREMENTS	
If you're mostly sedentary	0.7 grams/pound body weight
If you're a moderate exerciser	0.8 to 0.9 grams/pound body weight
If you're over 65; younger but have noticed muscle loss; or are an athlete or exercise vigorously	1 gram/pound body weight

TOP PROTEIN CHOICES	GRAMS PER 3-OUNCE SERVING (unless noted)
Chicken breast	26
Rib eye steak	25
Pork loin	23
Canned tuna	23
Shrimp	19
Halibut	19
Tempeh	17
Lamb	15
Tofu	15
Eggs (2 large)	13

WHERE ELSE TO GET PROTEIN	GRAMS
Lentils (1 cup)	18
Black beans (1 cup)	15
Chickpeas (1 cup)	15
Cottage cheese, 2% (½ cup)	12
Greek yogurt, low fat (½ cup)	11
Edamame (3 ounces)	10
Quinoa (1 cup)	8
Whole wheat spaghetti (1 cup)	7
Oatmeal (1 cup)	6
Green peas (½ cup)	4
Asparagus (1 cup)	4
Guava (1 cup)	4
Baked potato (1)	3

Coda: Thoughts on Weight Control, Intermittent Fasting, and Snacking

When we set about designing this Vital Sign, we had a few goals. One of the most important was to make it about what you *can* eat, not what you can't. There's a lot of obsessing over food these days, fear of eating certain types of food, even anxiety over whether certain basics like fruits and vegetables and meats are healthy *enough*. In many cases, this is misplaced precision. Eating doesn't have to be that hard. So we like to focus on what's in the eating plus column, rather than the minus column.

That isn't to say we are oblivious to the very real, widespread, and obstinate problem of obesity in our society, or that, closer to home, we don't work with people who want to lose weight. To the contrary. What we've found is that concentrating on the nutritious foods in this chapter's physical practice solves a lot of the overeating problems that lead to an unhealthy body weight. The foods are filling and mostly low or moderate in calories, and because there are no strict rules on the specific foods you need to choose or how to prepare them (frying being the only thing off-limits), you can select the ones you personally find the most satisfying. If you like pineapple, eat pineapple. If you find yams much more flavor-ful than your typical Idaho baked potato, go for it. Sauté your spinach in olive oil. Eat what you love. Our recommendations are flexible, and they're not going to leave you with a lot of room for sweets and chips and other danger-zone foods. If snacking is your downfall, you may even feel fine giving it up.

Snacking, in our opinion, can be highly overrated. Other cultures don't find it a necessity, yet the need to snack is ingrained in American society. Everyone's got an energy bar in their pocket, it seems. Then there's the idea that you need to snack to rev up your metabolism. Really, the key to weight loss is simply calories in and calories out, so even if eating bumps up your calorie burning a bit, does it do so enough to incinerate those snacking calories? This is a conundrum solved by only snacking when the stretch between meals is extralong or if you're having a small post-exercise protein snack.

As parents of two athletic daughters, we see a lot of oversnacking in kids' sports, and in fact we've lost a few parent friends who are horrified by our strong feelings about kids' overfueling. Kids don't need to be eat-ing at halftime during soccer or water polo games. And they definitely don't need the Doritos and donuts and other high-calorie foods that the "snack parents" bring to practices. We've asked Nic Gill, the strength and conditioning coach of the famed New Zealand rugby team, the All Blacks, what he thinks kids need at halftime while playing a sport that requires a lot of running. His answer was succinct: "A sip of water." A little more of our conversation:

"Do they need a post-workout meal?" we asked.

"Well, when's their game?"

"What if it's at nine in the morning?"

"Well, are they going to eat lunch?"

"I'm assuming they are."

"No, they don't need to eat a post-workout meal."

His point was that, if kids are eating a nutritious breakfast, lunch, and dinner, they don't need to be eating at halftime or right after a game. Very young kids, with their tiny stomachs, may need to eat more often than older kids. And yeah, we get that you're not going to be able to run errands with a toddler sans some Cheerios in your arsenal. But we'd argue that even toddlers are "oversnacked" these days. This isn't just about the immediate needs of kids; it also has to do with developing healthy habits and learning to eat when you're hungry, not just because food is available. There's also something to be learned here for adults as well. One is that when kids are fed constantly, they become adults who think they need to eat constantly. And adults, exercisers in particular, you don't need to eat constantly, not even to fuel your workouts. Fueling your way through a marathon is one thing, but that's very different from what we're seeing: "I'm going to my spin class. I have to eat first." No, you don't. "I need a sports drink to get me through a game of tennis." No, you don't. (Even Gatorade is on to this and has created a "zero sugar" drink.)

What we're asking you to do is reassess perhaps some of your long-held notions that you need to eat at various times. You really don't need to eat as often as you might think. Or drink. One of our strategies for keeping our weight stable is not drinking our calories (smoothies as meals excepted). We're not teetotalers; we can enjoy the celebratory alcoholic drink here and there. But to our mind, beverage calories can be better spent getting 800 grams of produce or meeting our daily protein needs.

As noted, we subscribe to the basic-healthy-eating method of maintaining a moderate weight, but what if you need to be more proactive? Any of the weight loss diets out there, provided they are based on nutritious foods and are sustainable, can work. If one suits your preferences and allows you to feel energetic and well nourished, we say go for it. These days a lot of people ask us about intermittent fasting (IF), the eating strategy that involves fasting for a certain number of hours each day or, a few days a week, eating just one meal. The theory behind IF is that going without food for a significant length of time encourages the body to burn fat and also decreases blood pressure and cholesterol. The cycling between fasting and eating is also said to prevent one of the typical adaptations of dieting, where the body, sensing deprivation, slows the metabolism in an effort to protect body weight.

If it works for you, great. But there are a few things to think about. In 2022, researchers reported in *The New England Journal of Medicine* that intermittent fasting had no benefits (one IF researcher, an IF devotee himself, was crushed by the news). Some research also suggests that IF may cause more muscle loss than other types of weight loss. While muscle forfeiture tends to be a casualty of any type of weight loss, a study led by researchers at the University of California, San Francisco, found that people who followed a 16:8 intermittent fasting diet (eating only within an eight-hour window, abstaining the other sixteen hours) experienced an unusual amount of muscle loss: 65 percent of the weight they took off was lean tissue—more than double what normally occurs. The researchers hypothesized that it may be because the IF dieters weren't getting enough protein.

As big fans of maintaining as much muscle as possible, that gives us pause. Intermittent fasting can be a slippery slope. If you're trying it, it's worth asking if it will allow you to get all the micro- *and* macronutrients you need. Ask yourself, too, why you're doing it. Fasting can be a really powerful tool to bring consciousness to your eating or give your gut a chance to take a break from digesting. But if you're starving yourself so you can go on vacation and look good in your suit, you're not really going to benefit long term.

What to Do When You Hurt

PAIN, LIKE DEATH AND TAXES, is part of the human condition. It's part of the human condition, too, to be able to triumph over pain—the body is an incredible healing machine. So as unpleasant and common as it is to feel musculoskeletal pain, don't freak out when you're hurting. Most times, musculoskeletal pain will dissipate on its own. If it doesn't, you usually have the ability to change, modify, attenuate, or eliminate it. Just adhering to the ten physical practices in this book will go a long way toward alleviating any aches you may have now and preventing pain and discomfort in the future. Moving more and being well rested, well fed, and less stressed out can also go a long way toward making your brain more tolerant and resilient to pain and discomfort. But when you need a first aid approach, here are some things to think about.

Pain is a request for change. Your brain gets input from the affected part of your body, then interprets that information as a threat or not, ultimately giving you the message that you need to do something differently. How differently depends. Pain doesn't always mean that you're injured or that a tissue is damaged; in fact, most times it doesn't. We define "injury" as a condition where there's obvious damage—a bone breaking the skin, an ankle swollen to the size of a tree branch—or the pain is unrelenting or such that you can't fulfill your typical role in life. If you can't care for your family, can't do your job, or are having what we call "red flags" like night sweats, fever, dizziness, nausea, or unaccounted-for weight loss or weight gain, you need to see your healthcare provider. Clear injury, pathology, or life-altering pain are all medical emergencies.

But most of the musculoskeletal pain people experience these days—

sore knees, achy lower backs, throbbing shoulders—is not injury, but rather a reflection of our modern lifestyle. It's rare, though, that people make the connection between poor sleep, not moving all day, limited range of motion, and congested tissues and the fact that their knees (or other parts) ache. The environment we live in is one where we drive everywhere, park ourselves in front of computers, pay other people to walk our dogs—many people don't even stroll the aisles of Costco anymore, now that you can get so many things delivered. The resulting disuse of various muscles and joints affects our movement ability, and yet it has been largely divorced from the conversation about pain.

When Kelly speaks to crowds, he'll often say, "Raise your hand if you're in pain," and a full 95 percent of the people—even when the audience includes fifteen-year-olds—shoot their hands into the air. It's no wonder, then, that many people are running to their doctors. According to a 2013 Mayo Clinic study, among the top reasons adults go to their primary care doctor is pain from arthritis, joint dysfunction, and back issues. The only thing that prompts more visits is skin problems.

We're not surprised that so many people turn to physicians and other healthcare practitioners for pain that isn't an obvious injury. No one tells them otherwise. If you go to a cycling class and you have nagging knee pain, the instructor is likely to suggest that you talk to a doctor or physical therapist. Where else are you going to turn? The elephant in the room is that people don't seek help soon enough. They deal with their discomfort until it gets so bad they are forced to confront it with a physician. Or they just deal with it by covering it up with pain medication, bourbon, THC, or any other thing that can stop the pain so that they can continue on the way they were. Might we suggest another solution?

Nothing against primary care doctors (Kelly is the son and grandson of physicians), but they aren't often well trained to look beyond obvious injury. In fact, the doctors we work with regularly complain that they simply don't have enough time to talk about the things that make up the contents of this book with their patients. It's like the system is set up to deal with pathology and catastrophe, not issues of lifestyle, tissue health, movement quality, and range of motion. So, when they can't find a specific diagnosis, they can offer you means to help manage the pain with pharmaceuticals, like nonsteroidal anti-inflammatory drugs (NSAIDs), opiates, or other medications. If you work out, they'll also usually give you some advice: Stop running, swimming, cycling, lifting—whatever it is you do, because it is causing you pain so severe you sought out a doctor (which is not unreasonable). For the person who gets real pleasure or stress relief from exercise, that can be soul killing. Physicians, for all they can do for us, have a limited toolbox when it comes to tender ankles and lower back pain. But you yourself actually have a very full toolbox for tending to body aches and pains. In fact, most times you can perform basic maintenance on yourself. You have the power to do simple things to make yourself feel better. Let's talk about how.

First Aid Kit

One thing you should know about your body is that it's not as fragile as you think. You are a pretty bombproof organism, easily designed to last a hundred years. That doesn't mean your body should hurt. It's actually normal for tissues to not hurt if you press on them; pressure should feel good, like a massage, or just like pressure. Why do they hurt sometimes? It could be any number of reasons. They're hypersensitized, overworked, or underhydrated, you under-slept, you ate too much pizza—we don't know. Could be anything. Follow the breadcrumbs and try to figure it out.

Upstream-Downstream Thinking

One of our favorite quotes comes from Ida Rolf, who developed the physical manipulation practice called Rolfing. Rolf, in her infinite wisdom, once said, "Whatever you think it is, it ain't." Less picturesque but equally salient is another quote we heard somewhere: "Where the rats get in is not where they chew."

What we're getting at is the fact that, when a body part hurts, it's often not because something is wrong with that body part, but rather that something is going on either below it (downstream) or above it (upstream). Knee pain, for instance, could be a symptom of stiff muscle and connective tissues of the quadriceps, hamstrings, or calves. An aching back might also originate with stiff quads or hamstrings, or maybe the butt. Your body is not just the sum of its parts; it's an interconnected system in which each element can have an effect on the others. We can't give you a diagnosis via book, but we can help you make a mental shift. Rather than just taking pain at face value, go look and see what else might be going on. Look upstream, then look downstream. Explore.

You have to freestyle a bit here. One way you can do that is to see what happens when you put some therapeutic pressure on an upstream or downstream body part. Try doing a series of contract-and-relax cycles on the associated spot in the offending position; better yet, do them in combination with input from a therapy ball or roller. Here are two examples of how to get a soothing input into an area so that it helps resolve your referred pain, which is the pain you feel in one part of your body that is actually caused by pain or injury in another part of your body. One note: When you use a foam roller, don't just move up and down on it. Moving side to side covers more of the "neighborhood," and by that we mean the nearby tissues. You can think of this like cutting a steak across the grain.

Pain Relief After Long-Duration Sitting

Remember when we talked about how you make a sort of panini out of your butt after you've been sitting for a long time (page 38)? Among other things, all the weight you put on those tissues messes up the blood flow and hydration of the tissue systems you are using as a chair. You may feel pain and stiffness in your back as a result. So here's a way to get things flowing properly again. You'll need a foam roller.

While seated on an armless chair or bench, place the end of a foam roller under one buttock so that your sit bone is parked firmly on top. Moving carefully so as not to lose your balance, roll your glutes and hamstrings side to side across the roller. Remember: We aren't just addressing the muscular system here. You may be giving input to the fascia of the glutes and low back as well. Keep rolling until you hit Switzerland—that is, it feels neutral, like nothing's happening anymore. Switch sides. Shoot for three to five minutes per leg. This is an example of mobilizing the tissues downstream of the low back and giving positional context to the mobilization (sitting).

Self-Soothe Painful Tissue

If an area of your body hurts when you press on the tissues, the contract/relax technique can help you desensitize that area. Contracting the tissues under the ball or roller might be more easily understood as creating nonthreatening input to the brain. This involves tightening up the muscles in the affected area—or the muscles upstream and downstream—for a few seconds, then relaxing them for a few seconds, and doing both in concert with your breathing. You can do this to any body part, but here's how you would do it for a sore knee using a ball or roller:

Lie facedown with a ball or roller under the quadriceps (upper thigh) of one leg. Inhale and contract your quadriceps for four seconds, then exhale and relax the muscle for eight seconds. Repeat the cycle until that hotspot begins to feel differently. In the clinic, we like to say: Mobilize until you make change, or until you stop making change.

To Ice or Not to Ice? There Is No Question

In 2012, we posted a video on YouTube titled "Icing Muscles Information." Here was the upshot: Don't ice sore or injured muscles. Ever. The backlash was swift and fierce (along the lines of "You can have my ice when you pry it from my cold, dead hands!"). People did not want to give up icing, and we can understand why. Cold numbs pain. Icing is what we've always been told to do. It's what our mom did, it's what we do for our kids when they bang their heads. It's always been accepted wisdom. And yet, while icing does effectively (if temporarily) relieve pain, it also does some other things, none of them good.

Just to clarify, we're not talking about the ice baths we describe on page 205. Icing an isolated, painful spot on the body is different. When there's trauma to a muscle, your goal should be to get it to heal fast, and the body actually has a very effective system for doing just that. The first order of business is to get rid of the damaged tissues and cells in and around the "accident" site, what physiologists call "waste." The second thing that has to happen is the regeneration of new muscle fibers and connective tissues. The body takes care of both tasks by sending in a repair-and-cleanup crew—only icing virtually stops that crew in its tracks by delaying the chemical signals that normally send them racing to the traumatized spot. With no removal imminent, the waste most often becomes trapped, and the area becomes congested. There is even evidence that when your tissues become numb under an ice bag, your lymphatic system becomes more porous. This means that all the waste that has already been sequestered gets reintroduced to the injured site. So what you do by applying cold in the service of quick relief creates a condition where healing is delayed or limited. Another thing to consider is that the inflammation that occurs after injury is not a bad thing. The inflammatory response is the driver of healing. It is not a mistake. That's one reason treating musculo-skeletal injuries with anti-inflammatories has also been called into question; in blocking pain it attenuates the healing response, too. Research is continuing in this area; meanwhile, the jury on anti-inflammatories like ibuprofen is still out.

Since the time we first broached the heresy of nixing icing in 2012, NOT icing has, in fact, begun to be regarded as best practice. Even the sports medicine physician Gabe Mirkin, who arguably started it all in a 1978 book by recommending injuries be treated with RICE (rest, ice, compression, elevation), no longer endorses icing. Research has been validating the retraction as well. In a 2021 animal study, a group of researchers from Kobe University and other institutions found that when mice (who have muscle tissue similar to humans') had their overexercised muscles iced, it took them longer to heal than non-iced mice. Looking at the muscles at the microscopic level, the researchers could see that it took the repair cells *four days* longer to reach the effective levels in the iced mice. Some research has also shown that icing can interfere with strength, endurance, and speed, so athletes in particular may want to give the ice pack a rest.

If cold is out, does that mean that heat is in? Heat is soothing and can indeed help with pain, especially when a muscle is spasming. Unlike cold, heat also increases circulation, which can speed healing. There are all kinds of ways to apply heat. A hot bath or shower. Hot tubs and saunas. Heating pads, hot-water bottles. You can even go top-of-the-line and get something like the Venom vibrating heat wrap. Low-tech or high-tech are equally good. If our goal is to soothe pain and not limit healing, heat wins over ice.

Because the sports world loves acronyms, there's another popular protocol now being recommended instead of RICE. It's called PEACE & LOVE and was outlined in the *British Journal of Sports Medicine* by researchers from Canada. Let us spell it out for you.

P Protect (avoid activities that increase pain the first few days after injury)

E Elevate (elevate the injured limb higher than your heart if possible)

A Avoid anti-inflammatories (anti-inflammatories and icing slow healing)

C Compress (use elastic bandages or tape to reduce swelling)

E Educate (avoid unnecessary passive treatments)

&

L Load (let your body tell you when it's safe to load again)

O Optimism (be confident and positive)

V Vascularization (choose cardio activities to get your heart rate up without causing pain)

E Exercise (take an active approach to recovery)

SQUAT!

ASSESSMENT
Squat Test

PHYSICAL PRACTICE
Squatting Variations

WHEN WAS THE last time you organized your body into a full squat, bending your knees deeply and dropping your butt low to the ground? Maybe it was at the gym this morning. Maybe it was the last time you had to get down to see eye to eye with a three-year-old. In Western culture, squatting is considered either a strengthening exercise or a necessity on the rare occasion we need to talk to a toddler. And yet to squat is to arrange yourself into an innately human position. Our bodies are built to squat, and in many cultures it's as common as sitting in a chair.

In 2018, *The Atlantic* published an article about what it called "the Asian squat," accompanied by photos of people squatting while taking photos, eating, smoking (not recommended!), waiting for customers, looking at art—you get the drift. Not shown, but well known, is the fact that many Asians still use squat toilets. Some women give birth in this position, too. We were wowed by how effortlessly the people whose photos graced *The Atlantic* could squat—one of them was the prime minister of Singapore, and he was wearing a suit.

Although we are not what you'd call a squatting culture, all of us do a modified squat many, many times a day without even realizing it. Every time you get in and out of a chair, every time you get on and off the toilet, you are actually doing a midrange squat. All we're asking you to do here is to take it further, into a full-range squat, the kind the prime minister of Singapore was photographed so elegantly illustrating. We're talking about going all the way down into a position you can hang out in. If you lower yourself into a chair several times a day and, of course, if you're doing workout squats, you're already halfway there or more.

Various positions take different joints to their normal end ranges. That's why, for example, we have you doing mobilizations for hip extension (Vital Sign 3) and shoulder rotation (Vital Sign 5). The squat is one of the rare positions that allows you to practice several normal ranges: hip flexion and external rotation, knee flexion, and ankle dorsiflexion. It's the actual expression of what every range-of-motion chart used by every orthopedic surgeon and physical therapist says those joints should be able to do, but all at once. To some of you, squatting may seem hard but, again, it's what nature designed your body to do.

There are a few tangible things that happen when you improve your squatting ability. One is helping you avoid lower back pain. When you're lacking hip flexion, you end up using your lumbar spine to solve movement problems that your hip should solve for you. Say you bend over to pull weeds in your garden or are at the airport and must bend over to pick up your luggage. These are things you might do on repeat as you move from one area of the garden to another or relocate from the ticket counter to airport security to the snack shop. If you can't effectively squat to make these transitions, you must round your back to bend over, introducing inefficiency to your movement system (your hips are much stronger than your spine and better at bigger ranges of motion under load).

So that's one reason being able to squat is a good thing. Squatting also allows you to practice good ankle range of motion, which in turn will help with balance and the ankle's ability to weather trouble. When your brain knows that it's okay for the ankle to go to its end range, your body can make quick adjustments to stay steady on uneven ground and when coming down from a lay-up. And if you do turn your ankle? You're more likely to walk away unscathed because your ankle was able to move as it should.

Squatting is something we did naturally as children; as adults, it can feel challenging if you haven't done it for a while. The following assessment will provide a good starting point for those of you who need to work on the position. For those of you who find sinking your center of gravity, ass to ankle, a snap, it'll be a good reminder that you need to go there on a regular basis so that those four main ranges—hip flexion and rotation, knee flexion, ankle dorsiflexion—stay well within your capability.

Assessment: Squat Test

We think everyone should be able to squat with their feet parallel and in reference foot position (toes straight ahead, weight balanced between the balls and the heels of the feet) and hip crease below the knee. We're not so stringent that we insist your torso must be upright (that's a different move, suitable for doing squat exercises). Your torso can come forward and, in fact, it will help you stay balanced as you squat. Believe it or not, once you get used to it, it can actually be a fairly comfortable position to hang out in.

If this all sounds impossible, let us assure you that most people can ultimately get there. Let's see where you are now; then we'll tell you about how you can work toward conquering the squat.

PREPARATION
You'll need some clear floor space. Wear nonrestricting clothes and, if you like, shoes, though barefoot is okay, too.

THE TEST

Before you take the test, a note about the positioning of your back. When you're holding something heavy (like a weight) in a squat, it's optimal to keep your back straight and torso upright. But when you're just squatting without any encumbrances, it doesn't matter if your back is straight. In fact, when you are in a deep squat and allow your back to round, it's very restorative for the spine, helping to rehydrate the disks. So don't worry about your back during this test; concentrate on your hips and feet. Here's what to do:

Stand straight with your feet hip width or farther apart. It doesn't matter how wide your stance is, and a wider stance may make it easier to squat, so choose what feels right. Next, bend your knees and lower your butt toward the ground, keeping your feet straight, your weight balanced between your heels and the balls of your feet. Place your arms out in front of you and lean your torso forward if it helps you maintain balance. Don't worry about the shape of your spine as you squat. Now try to achieve one of these squat positions. Whatever position you reach, hold it for five breaths:

1 The ideal position you're aiming for is butt a few inches above the floor, hip crease well below the knees, toes pointed forward, heels flat on the floor.

2 If you can't reach the first position without falling, try angling your toes outward and separating your legs farther apart, or keeping your feet straight ahead but allowing your heels to rise (if you can manage it, this is preferable to the toes-angled-outward position).

3 If this is still too difficult, try to lower your hips to the height of a chair seat so your legs form about a 90-degree angle.

4 As a last alternative, lower your hips as far as they will go.

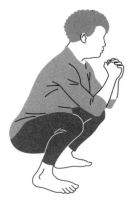

We've never seen a child that doesn't spend lots of time playing in this position. Our goal: Reclaim our youthful movement. YES, it's possible.

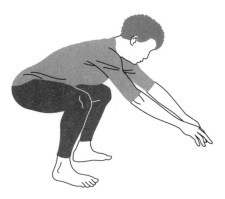

Turning your feet out is a fine way to achieve depth in your squat but may limit your movement choice and power.

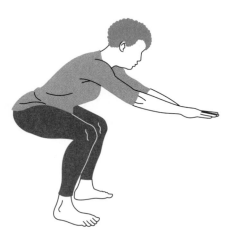

Note that this squat height corresponds to a chair level. Coincidence?

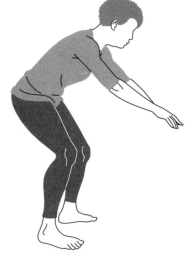

It's not where you start; it's where you end! Keep it up!

WHAT YOUR RESULTS MEAN

If you reached position 1: You're a ninja! This is good news in terms of your hip, knee, and ankle range of motion. As per our usual recommendation, don't take your squat prowess for granted. You can skip the Sit-Stands in the physical practice (page 203), but practice hanging out in a deep squat at least three times a week.

If you reached position 2: You're almost there. Keeping your feet facing forward is the most challenging element of squatting. Many people can do a deep squat with their feet angled out, which is fine—but when your feet are angled, the position allows you to hide deficiencies in ankle and hip range of motion and doesn't lend itself to maintaining a stable arch in the foot. That's why it's worth trying to improve your foot position. However, what's most important is that you, like the people who hit position 1, make squatting a regular part of your health regimen, feet angled or straight.

If you reached position 3: Just being able to lower to chair height and hold it is notable. As you work the Vital Sign 7 physical practice, you will gradually be able to drop below this 90-degree angle.

If you reached position 4: This is obviously an arduous move for you, but we've never seen anyone who can't master the squat. The physical practice we have in store will let you gradually improve at a reasonable pace.

WHEN SHOULD YOU RETEST?

If you're able to do a deep squat, you can test daily, because we recommend hanging out in that position every day. If you're not able to squat and are following the Sit-Stand protocol (page 203), test once a week until you master the deep squat. After that, you can just retest every day in your Deep Squat Hang-Out.

The Low Down

The very first video we ever posted on YouTube was called "The 10-Minute Squat Test." That was way back in 2010, filmed in our old backyard—we just pointed the camera at Kelly as he squatted (and talked) for ten minutes, explaining the benefits of what he was doing and how to squat in a way that would maximize range of motion in the hips, ankles, and knees. As professional athletes, we had traveled quite a bit by then and had seen people squatting all over the world (and used a few squatty potties ourselves). But we knew that very few people back home ever engineered their body into this all-important shape—many of them couldn't do it if they tried. We wanted to change that, and for good reason.

We'd wager that there is not a physician in the country who advises their patients to squat for good health. And yet there's evidence that squatting really can make a difference in your well-being. Researchers at Chinese and U.S. universities collaborated in 2002 to publish the results of a study comparing the prevalence of arthritis of the hip in elderly people in China and the United States. The study found that the occurrence of arthritic hip pain in Chinese men and women was *80 to 90 percent* lower than for their American counterparts. Some of the difference could probably be attributed to genetics, but some of it, concluded the researchers, was also attributable to the way the Chinese use their bodies on a daily basis. Here's what the researchers wrote: "Squatting utilizes an extreme range of motion that may engage areas of hip cartilage that are not loaded during upright stance, possibly stimulating turnover and regeneration of cartilage that is otherwise subject to disuse-related thinning and more vulnerable to stress."

When you're squatting, two other joints are also in play: the ankles and the knees. The ankle in particular is underappreciated. This evolutionary gift of nature is critical to maintaining balance, something we'll go into further in Vital Sign 8. Equally important, your ankles help you get up from the ground. If you have good range of motion in the ankles, you'll likely ace the Sit-and-Rise Test in Vital Sign 1, which also means you'll be able to get up if you fall. Athletes benefit when ankles have proper mobility, too. Having full range of motion in your ankles allows you to put more power into dynamic moves like running, jumping, taking lateral steps, and pushing off the side of a pool wall. (Athletic types should also note that the hip flexion practiced in squatting will improve your cycling power.) And, to reiterate, ankles with good mobility protect against injury, too.

The other joint of consequence here is the knee joint. There's an old idea that squatting below a 90-degree angle is bad for your knees. You wouldn't hesitate to bend your elbow at 90 degrees. The joints are designed to bend deeply, knee joints included. Far from hurting the knees, squatting helps strengthen the muscles that support them, and in fact one of the most human of all processes depends on the ability to squat with the knees in a deep bend—or at least it used to. We're talking about pooping. Something that gets little airtime—understandably so, since no one really wants to talk about pooping—is that in cultures where people squat to toilet, there is a lower incidence of digestive diseases like irritable and inflammatory bowel syndromes. Squatting is the natural position for this most natural of bodily functions. The toilet, like the chair and the smartphone and the computer and the car . . . and on and on . . . is another modern convenience that doesn't quite square with the design of our bodies. Are we asking you to give it up? Of course not—that ship has sailed—but we think it further drives home the point that squatting is a normal position that we should be adopting regularly.

So, okay, unless you're traveling or camping, you're probably not going to be squatting to toilet, but you will undoubtedly at some time need to pick something up off the floor. Here's where being able to squat comes in really handy. If needed, you can bend over at a 90-degree angle at your hips with your back flat and legs straight. But what if you need to go lower? How do you get to the ground? There are essentially two choices. You can hinge with your knees bent and pick up that toy or bag of laundry, but you'll need to employ the smaller muscles of your back to do so instead of the big muscles of your legs. Your other choice is to go into a deep squat, which not only gets you down low but also allows you to drive out of that bottom shape using your legs and butt (largest muscles in the body) to power you and that box of old cookware up and out to the garage. This is the safer and more efficient option, and it gives you the opportunity to practice various ranges of motion to boot.

WARMING UP FOR EXERCISE

We're often asked if mobilizations, including rolling exercises, are a good warmup for working out. The short answer is yes, with a caveat. If you're doing a sport or workout that requires full range of motion in a joint (and they mostly all do), it's not going to go as well as it might otherwise if you have limited range of motion. So, for instance, if you're going to be running, you might include the Couch Stretch (page 94) in your warmup, because it puts your body into a position—hip extension—that you'll use in running. For the same reason, swimmers should warm up with shoulder mobility exercises. The problem is, we often see people using mobilizations, especially soft tissue mobilizations with rolling, that don't fit the sport they're prepping for. Rolling out your calves won't help your kayaking strokes. Plus, would you have a massage before getting on your bike or stepping into a boxing ring? Definitely use mobilizations to warm up, but use the ones that improve the positions you'll be using in your activity of choice.

The other part of warming up is, well, warming up. You need to get hot and at least a little sweaty to prime your muscles for movement. To us, the perfect tool for that is the jump rope. Jumping rope, or even doing the modified version—bouncing—for two to five minutes is great prep for any kind of workout, and it's an excellent way to improve balance (more on this in Vital Sign 8). Two for the price of one effort. If you're jump/bounce averse, just do some brisk walking. That will be enough to warm you up for your main activity.

As you go through the warmup process, also use it as a chance to assess how you're feeling on a given day. Kelly had an opportunity to fly in a plane with the Blue Angels, the U.S. Navy flight demonstration squadron that does acrobatics in the sky. One of the things he observed was how the pilots prepare for their virtuoso aerial moves. Once their planes are loaded up and in the air, the pilots do some high-speed turns to see how the plane feels fully loaded and how their bodies are going to handle the G-forces that day. Their susceptibility to the forces generated by the aircraft is predicated on many things, including hydration and sleep and just personal tolerance; they're doing a systems check.

Just like the Blue Angels, all of us are subject to variations in how well we are equipped to handle a particular endeavor. A pre-workout warmup is like a pilot's systems check: an assessment of how you're feeling that day. How tired are you? How stiff or springy do you feel? Does anything hurt? Use your warmup time to answer these questions, then proceed accordingly.

Physical Practice: Squatting Variations

Even if you can't remember ever squatting, you likely did so as a young child. And your body remembers, even if it doesn't seem to like it at first. It's like the pipes have already been laid; you just have to turn on the faucet. It's a skill that's shockingly recoverable.

Remember as you go through this physical practice that you're not just improving your squatting technique for its own sake. You use squatting movements all the time. For instance, if you lose your balance, you end up defaulting to a single-leg squat to try to catch yourself. Going up and down the stairs is a single-leg squat. So besides taking several different joints to their end ranges, what you're practicing when you squat is the root language of getting up and down.

Sit-Stands

These moves provide a way to gradually retrain your body to feel comfortable in a deep squat. They start with a chair as a support, then help you progress to prop-free squatting.

Stand with the back of your legs near the back of a chair. Holding your arms straight out at shoulder height, slowly bend your knees and lower your butt down onto the chair seat as if to sit, touch for a second, then slowly rise back up. Take two to three seconds to lower down and don't plop into the chair. On day one, do this once. On day two, do two in a row. On day three, do three in a row. Keep adding one squat each day until you reach twenty. Now lower your squat. Repeat the same sequence, but instead of a chair, use something lower, such as an ottoman or coffee table. When you reach twenty, repeat the sequence, lowering all the way into a deep squat.

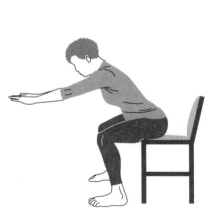

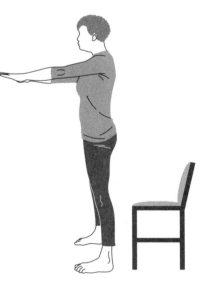

Keep your foot pressure even from the balls of your feet to your heels. Let your body move as it needs to keep your foot pressure even throughout.

No need to linger in the squat. Just lower slowly, then rise back up at a similar pace.

Deep Squat Hang-Outs

The best way to tell your brain you value something is to spend time in that position. If you have already mastered the deep squat, you just need to spend some time—even just three minutes a day—in the position to ensure that you don't lose the ability. You can drop it into your movement breaks during your workday or insert it into the time you spend sitting on the floor (Vital Sign 1) in the evenings as you watch TV.

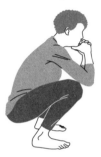

Strive to spend some time each day in this position.

EXTRA CREDIT: TABATA SQUATS

Way back in the 1990s, a Japanese physician and researcher popularized an intermittent training technique that became known as Tabata. The protocol goes like this: repeating cycles of twenty seconds of work, ten seconds of rest, for four minutes. This type of training improves the cardiovascular system as well as strength and endurance. If you're crushing the Deep Squat Hang-Outs, give it a try:

Stand with your feet shoulder-width apart in reference foot position (toes pointing straight ahead, weight balanced between the balls and heels of your feet). Bend your knees and squat, allowing your hip crease to drop well below your knees. Rise up and repeat the squat as many times as you can in twenty seconds. Rest for ten seconds. Do eight cycles, or as many as possible in four minutes. Count your reps with each twenty-second cycle. Your "score" is the lowest number of squats in a cycle. Work toward getting all cycles up to your highest number of squats.

A STUDY IN CONTRAST: HOT AND COLD THERAPY

One of the best investments we ever made was putting a little sauna in our backyard. The next best investment was getting a cold plunge bath and placing it right next to the sauna. This way we can heat up, then cool down, and repeat, a process known as "contrast therapy." Obviously, contrast therapy gets the first part of its name from the polar-opposite temperatures you're exposed to when you jump back and forth from a heat source to a cold source. The "therapy" part is the good stress it puts on the body: It's like a workout for the vascular system, constricting and expanding the blood vessels so more blood is pumped throughout, delivering greater loads of oxygen and nutrients to the muscles. Same with the lymphatic channels; they get "pumped," too. We use contrast therapy to help speed up recovery from the natural breakdown of muscle tissue from exercise, so there's less soreness and faster adaptation to the exertion we've put our bodies through earlier in the day.

You don't have to have a sauna to do contrast therapy—or a dedicated cold plunge tub—but we like the sauna for its own benefits. Among them: lowering the risk of high blood pressure, cardiovascular disease, stroke, and Alzheimer's, and successful treatment of arthritis, headache, and flu. Regular sauna-ing also improves immune function, so it can help you avoid getting sick in the first place. Spend five to twenty minutes in a sauna at 80 to 100 degrees Fahrenheit and you'll reap the rewards. Those Finns aren't healthy for nothing.

Cold immersion has its own perks. We're not talking about icing an injury. That's a different kettle of fish, and not recommended (see page 190). One—icing an injury—prevents inflammatory cells from aiding in the healing of tissue in need of repair. The other—cold immersion— reduces the lower-grade inflammation that's associated with muscles that have worked hard. Cold immersion has been around for a long time, but has been most recently popularized by Wim Hof (see page 68), known for his legendary feats of endurance in the cold and advocacy of cold-water showers and baths. As Hof has noted, exposure to cold water is linked to improved immune and cardiovascular function as well as better sleep. In 2016, Brazilian researchers compared the results of nine studies on cold-water immersion and found that it improved muscle recovery at a dose of eleven to fifteen minutes at a temperature of 50 to 59 degrees Fahrenheit.

Contrast therapy is something you might need to dip a toe into first—that is, take it slow. You'll find that both temperatures can increase your heart rate and speed up your breathing, which is normal but can be anxiety-provoking at first. Start small, especially with the cold part of the contrast, even just putting a limb or two in at first; then work up to longer, full-body sessions (most people find that heat takes less time than cold to get used to). There are all different ways to do it, including just using your shower's temperature controls.

Our own personal protocol for contrast therapy goes like this: We spend about fifteen minutes in the sauna, then cold plunge for three minutes, and repeat the rotation several times. Besides how great we feel afterward, one of the things we love about it is that it's turned into a bit of a social hour at our house. We'll invite friends over for dinner, then end the evening with a sauna and cold plunge cycle. It's a lot healthier than a nightcap and gets everyone a little sleepy (we end with a session in the cold plunge since it helps bring the core temperature down in a way that prepares the body for sleep). We all rest really well that night.

FIND YOUR BALANCE

ASSESSMENT
PART 1: SOLEC (Stand On One Leg, Eyes Closed) Test;
PART 2: Old Man Balance Test

PHYSICAL PRACTICE **Balance Exercises and Mobilizations**

AFTER JULIET GRADUATED from college, she moved a lot of her things into a storage unit. Among the things she warehoused was a potted succulent that had previously enjoyed lots of California sun, as well as Juliet's TLC. When she went to move out of the storage unit, Juliet found the once thriving plant, starved of water and light for more than a year, seemingly dead. "What the hell," she thought, "I might as well try watering it"—only to see the withered succulent spring back to life. It turned back on.

That's what we're trying to do in this chapter: Turn your ability to balance back on. Even if it seems diminished, it's ripe for resuscitation. Although maybe you don't think this applies to you. Maybe you walk around fine, never tripping and falling. Okay—the assessments we've got coming up for you will reveal the truth. But everyone, no matter how steady on their feet right now, needs to practice balance. For safety, for the confidence to do what you want and need to do without fear, for easier movement, for fewer aches and pains, and for better athletic performance. There really are innumerable reasons.

Of all the many physical competencies we possess, balance is the unsung hero, the attribute that's on few people's radars but affects just about every aspect of mobility. Perhaps we shouldn't say it isn't on *anyone's* radar. As people get into their sixties and above, they start hearing warnings about the dangers of loss of balance. And this is indisputably a true worldwide problem, and the numbers in the United States alone are disturbing. According to the CDC, every second of every day, an older adult falls—that's about 36 million falls a year, and it's the leading cause of injury and injury-related death in older people. The fallout from falling also extends to people leading smaller lives, restricting themselves from activities and social interactions, and ultimately moving less, getting weaker, and impairing their balance even more, a detrimental loop.

In some ways, society accepts this as just the price of aging, but we reject that passive view. We know that falls don't always have to happen and that balance can be retained—and regained. Not incidentally, the very notion that falling is only a problem facing older people is wrong. A long line of researchers has looked at falls in younger people, including a group at Purdue University that found, within the confines of a four-month study, that half of the college-aged students surveyed fell down. *Every* student averaged a trip or slip per week, though most times they were able to catch themselves before falling. A small percentage of the falls were attributed to substance abuse (this was college, after all), and there were some falls while texting. But the biggest factor in falls was talking to someone else while walking. Lest you think this is something that only happens to head-in-the-clouds college students, there are also some sobering statistics: Falls are the third leading cause of unintentional injuries for people ages eighteen to thirty-five years old.

We know all this sounds a little doom and gloom, but it's actually just the opposite. Being upright in gravity is such a human thing, there's no reason your balance has to diminish. If everyone paid attention to balance right now, we feel certain those dire fall numbers would drop steeply. And by paying attention to balance we don't mean formal training that's going to take an hour out of your day. Improving balance isn't onerous—you can do it while brushing your teeth or washing the dishes—and it's a lot like play, which, since you presumably were once a kid, you already know how to do well. This is one place where you can see a massive difference with just a small amount of effort. Suddenly, the person who couldn't stand on one leg for twenty seconds is balancing on a slackline, then balancing on a slackline with their eyes closed, then juggling on a slackline . . . Okay, we're exaggerating, but just a bit. You really can make headway!

Assessment: Part 1: SOLEC (Stand On One Leg, Eyes Closed) Test; Part 2: Old Man Balance Test

There are various ways to measure balance. We chose these two particular tests because they assess different elements of the ability: The SOLEC Test takes visual information out of the equation, and the Old Man Balance Test gauges dynamic balance—can you balance while in motion? Both tests will also tell you a lot about your feet, which are intimately connected to balance. If your feet are well organized and sensitized enough to send information to your brain, chances are you'll score well on these tests.

Part 1: SOLEC (Stand On One Leg, Eyes Closed) Test

How steady you are on your feet depends—besides on your feet themselves—on three main factors: your inner ear; sensory receptors in the muscles, tendons, fascia, and joints; and eyesight. Your eyes help you stay steady by telling you where your body is in relation to your surroundings. Without the ability to see, you must depend on your body's other balance tools; this test measures how well those tools are working. It will also give you a sense of how integral vision is to maintaining balance—it's not easy to stand on one leg with your eyes closed. And yet it just takes a little training to become proficient at this difficult task.

PREPARATION

Because you'll be doing this test with your eyes closed, it's best to have someone help you do the timing. You'll need a watch or clock with a second hand, a place on the floor clear of any items, and bare feet.

THE TEST

Stand barefoot on the floor in an open, uncluttered space. Close your eyes, bend one leg, and raise your foot off the floor as high as comfortable (it doesn't need to go high). Stay in this position for twenty seconds, counting the number of times you touch your foot down. Switch sides. If you feel uneasy, stand next to a wall or in front of a sink.

Your arms don't have to be crossed. Not using your arms to balance is more difficult.

WHAT YOUR RESULTS MEAN

Your score is the number of times you touched the floor with your foot to regain balance. Assess each side separately.

You didn't touch at all—This is an indication that you have good mastery of balance. Practicing the test every day may be all the physical practice you need to maintain it.

You touched one to two times—Pretty good. This test will likely be a piece of cake for you with a little practice.

You touched three or more times—You've come to the right place. Your balance needs work, so pay close attention to everything you learn in this chapter.

WHEN SHOULD YOU RETEST?

There's no reason you can't take this test every day—taking the test is a balance practice in itself.

Part 2: Old Man Balance Test

We owe this simple, but telling, assessment to Chris Hinshaw, a renowned endurance coach and founder of aerobiccapacity.com. Don't let the name of the test fool you: It isn't easy for anyone, young or old. Nonetheless, we wouldn't include it in the book if we didn't think everyone can pass it with practice. And since mobility interacts with balance to help you master it, all the other practices you're doing will help you get that eventual A.

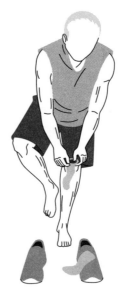

PREPARATION

You'll need a wide-open place on the floor, clear of any items, and bare feet. Place a pair of lace-up shoes and socks on the floor in front of you.

THE TEST

Balancing on your right leg, allow the left leg to extend behind you as you reach down to pick

The shoe game is really just about slipping skills into your daily routine. You are going to put shoes and socks on for the rest of your life. That's a ton of repetition!

up one shoe. Return to an upright position. Without holding on to anything if you can help it, raise your left foot and put on your sock, then reach down, pick up your shoe and put it on. Tie your shoe, then return your left foot to the floor. Repeat on the other side. Remember to breathe as you are balancing.

WHAT YOUR RESULTS MEAN

Your score is the number of times you touched the floor with your foot to regain balance. Assess each side separately.

> **You didn't touch at all**—This is an indication that you have good mastery of balance. Practicing the test every day may be all the physical practice you need to maintain it.
> **You touched one to two times**—Pretty good. This test will likely be a piece of cake for you with a little practice.
> **You touched three or more times**—You've come to the right place. Your balance needs work, so pay close attention to everything you learn in this chapter.

WHEN SHOULD YOU RETEST?

There's no reason you can't take this test every day—taking the test is a balance practice in itself.

Balance, from Head to Toe

If you watch a baby develop over the course of several months, you can see them exploring, then mastering balance. It starts with trying to right themselves as they learn to sit up, then advances as they begin to stand on two feet and cruise around. Even then, it takes them time to become proficient. You might remember the study we mentioned on page 35: Researchers observed that twelve- to nineteen-month-olds fell an average of seventeen times per hour. But falling when you weigh 25 pounds versus falling when you weigh 125 or 225 pounds is far less impactful. (That's why we try to be really good at *not* falling.) Judging from how often toddlers get up and try again, it barely impacts them at all.

All this is to say that balance is something that, early in life, we have to work at. Yet once we conquer it, we tend to ignore it, even though working at it—if only a little bit—is something we should do throughout our lifespan. Perhaps one reason we don't is that balance is a complex system, involving many different "tools" in many different places in the body. Most people don't even know what allows us to stay steady on our feet. So let's review.

Balance depends on an interchange of information between sensory elements and mechanical elements in the body. The brain integrates data from sources all the way down at your feet all the way up to your eyes to enable you to stay stable without even thinking about it. It's data processing power at the fastest, highest level designed to keep your head up and body safe so you can eat and reproduce and do all the things humans are supposed to do.

There are three main systems involved in the interplay of sensation and reaction. One of them is the vestibular system, otherwise known as the inner ear, a labyrinth of ring-shaped canals and tiny organs filled with fluid, each sensitive to different types of motion. When the head moves, the fluid in these structures moves with it, agitating minuscule hair cells that then transmit impulses to the brain. The brain subsequently directs the body to respond in order to maintain equilibrium.

We also rely heavily on another system, called "proprioception." Embedded in the muscles, joints, ligaments, and tendons are receptors that send information about the body's position and movements to the central nervous system, which then signals the muscles to properly respond—in fact, the whole point of having a central nervous system (the dual processing center of the brain and spinal cord) is to allow us to perceive changes in the environment, orient ourselves, and move competently to maintain our center of gravity. And not just competently, but quickly. The time between sensory input and protective muscle movement is just milliseconds. In this way, proprioception helps you make adjustments that allow you to right yourself when you trip on a rug and regain balance on a bike when you start to waver. It also helps basketball players dribble the ball without looking down and soccer players execute a kick without falling. In the blink of an eye, proprioception gives you incisive body awareness. Close your eyes and touch the top of your head. That's proprioception at work, too.

Everything, though, works better with your eyes open because vision is the third arm of the balance triad. When the head moves, the inner ear signals the eyes to move in ways that stabilize the gaze. Without this steadiness of sight, it would be difficult to avoid the obstacles that can cause us to lose our balance. But it's also more nuanced than that. As you can see by taking the SOLEC Test, it's difficult to maintain equilibrium when you subtract sight from the balance system. Even if you're not really moving, your eyes provide the brain with information that helps you stay upright.

Note that word "information," because that really is the key to balance. The brain is dependent on intel from various places within the body; without it, things literally get shaky. This is a good place to bring the feet into the conversation. We talked about how important the feet are in relation to walking (Vital Sign 4); in regard to balance, they warrant further discussion. Leonardo da Vinci said, "The human foot is a masterpiece of engineering and a work of art." He got that right. Beyond the fact that the feet are the foundation upon which our whole body weight sits, the feet have so much to tell us. Proprioceptors are particularly concentrated in the soles of the feet, and there is a lot of real estate in the brain devoted to information sent from the feet—about as much space as devoted to interpreting what the hands have to say.

Because most people rarely go barefoot, primarily walk on smooth surfaces, and stuff their feet into cushy shoes—the human movement specialist Phillip Beach calls shoes "sensory deprivation chambers"; Kelly refers to them as "coffins"—they're robbed of a lot of the input that helps build balance. There may be other consequences, too. One of the hypotheses out there is that some people may have back pain because of a lack of information coming up the chain about where they are in space. Without sufficient data, the brain starts to make poor judgments about how the body should be organized and move, potentially leading to discomfort and loss of function.

To contribute to balance in the way they're meant to, the feet need to be both strong and super sensitive to stimuli—it's not for nothing that some NFL teams have their players run barefoot from time to time. If you're a movie buff, you might remember that in the original *Die Hard* film (1988), Bruce Willis's character, John McClane, is advised by his seatmate that the secret to air travel is to take off your shoes and socks after you reach your destination, walk around barefoot, and make fists with your toes. It's actually sage advice, although it doesn't go so well for McClane, who, due to unforeseen circumstances, ends up spending the whole movie shoeless.

The ankles have an important role to play in balance, too. Like the feet, they have a high concentration of sensors for letting the brain know where you are in space. The ankles also must have a good range of motion (see page 199) so they can dexterously respond to things underfoot, like rocks on a trail or shifting sand on a beach, that threaten to topple us over. We like to say that the mark of a really good skier is not that they don't ever lose their balance but that they recover so well. It is pretty normal for your balance to be challenged; it's how well you can manage it that's at issue. When your ankles have good range of motion, your brain knows it and acts accordingly, sending signals that enable you to quickly recover when elements in the environment challenge your balance.

ARCH COMMENTARY

The arch of the foot is golden. A small structure built of bones, fascia, ligaments, and tendons, it helps balance the body's weight between the heel and the ball of the foot and it turns the foot into a springy, dynamic platform from which a zillion different moves can be launched. The medical establishment thinks the arch is so critical that artificial arch supports (orthotics) have even been developed to put into shoes.

Everyone agrees the arch is important. But to paraphrase the great running coach Nicholas Romanov, if you look at a bridge with an arch—google the New River Gorge Bridge in West Virginia, or one of the many arch bridges in China—you can see what's holding up the arch: nothing. Well, not entirely nothing. The weight of an arch structure is carried outward to the sides, called "abutments," and, in the case of the foot, the heel and ball. What we're getting at is that the arch should be more or less self-supporting. There may be times when some artificial support is warranted due to injury or extreme foot pain, but to wear arch supports for life is like spraining your arm and continuing to wear a sling when it heals. The support aid isn't only unnecessary; it impedes the strengthening of the structure so that it stays weak. Our opinion is that if you want to shut down the foot for good, give it an arch support—then it doesn't have to do any work.

Even people with so-called flat feet or "collapsed arches" have functional arches, although many of them think they don't. We can ask a roomful of people to get into the reference foot position (page 120) and suddenly some of them discover that the arches they always thought were nonexistent were just hiding in plain sight. Granted, some people have very low arches, but in all the feet we've surveyed, we've never detected one person who didn't have an arch that was apparent when they stood in reference foot position. What this means is that simply organizing your body better will improve the functionality of your arches, which will translate into more spring in your step and better balance.

It will also help you avoid "collapsed feet," which is entirely different from collapsed arches. Collapsed feet occur when the weight is not evenly distributed between the front and back of your feet and your ankles lean in toward each other. Limited ankle range of motion can contribute to collapsed feet, and the condition is often a harbinger of lower leg injury.

A while back we worked with a Division I women's swim team, and one of the things we were trying to do was help the athletes strengthen their ankles and feet. Most of the women, when out of the water, were wearing either flip-flops or super soft shoes with arch support, which had left their feet weak and desensitized. Strengthening their feet, we reasoned, would give them a more powerful push off the wall and get them off the starting blocks faster. During the first two weeks of foot-centric conditioning—which involved reorganizing their foot position while standing and walking and training on balance blocks—we were getting texts from the swimmers complaining about how their feet were cramping as they walked around campus. Never mind that they were superstar athletes—their feet were weak! But after the first two weeks, the cramping stopped and they began to see dividends in the pool. Even their kicking improved, because they were seeing better function up the whole chain.

Balancing Acts

Juliet's mom, Janet, swore off bike riding when she was in her sixties, feeling uncertain about whether she could balance on two wheels. We'd go on vacation with her and would want to rent bikes and she was like, "Nope." She's now seventy-seven, and although she's been a lifelong exerciser, is very fit, lean, and vibrant, and has now taken up dance and tai chi—both of which are great for fortifying balance—she's yet to get back up on a bike. Like most people, Janet just didn't know that she needed to pay attention to balance when she was younger, and her regular pursuits didn't have a balance-bolstering dividend.

There is a direct association between Janet's trepidation toward bike riding and our own avid mountain biking practices—we want to do everything we can to make sure it doesn't happen to us. We also have in mind the example of someone of approximately the same age as Juliet's mom, Bob Licht, who's the founder of Sea Trek sea kayaking adventures. Bob still stand-up paddles, whitewater kayaks, and mountain bikes. He can because he's been doing it for years. Neither Bob nor Janet is good or bad; they're just good examples of what can happen with balance. As with so many things, balance is a use-it-or-lose-it proposition.

We won't argue with the fact that the body is subject to change with age. In the balance realm, certain things do occur. When we get older, the central nervous system doesn't integrate the various signals it gets from our balance apparatus as well or as quickly. The functioning of proprioception receptors declines. Changes occur in the inner ear, particularly among those impulse-transmitting hair cells, which diminish. And, of course, most people don't see as well as the years go by (although somewhat paradoxically, and probably due to proprioception decline, we depend more on vision for balance as we age). All these things—even without the complicating factors of conditions like arthritis and diabetes, which can affect the feet and ankles—come together to make it more difficult to stay steady in the face of balance challenges.

There's some inevitability here, "some" being the operative word. There is good evidence to suggest (and not just of the Bob Licht variety) that exercise and balance training can stem some of the natural deterioration of the balance systems. For instance, proprioception, which probably contributes the most to balance at all ages, has been shown to improve in people who regularly do tai chi. Way back in 1997, a study at the Western University of Ontario found that, while younger people (ages nineteen to twenty-seven) definitely had more finely tuned proprioception than older people (ages sixty to eighty-six), older people who exercised had better proprioception than older people who did not.

The people in that Canadian study didn't specifically work on balance. So, what happens if you do? In 2020, a group of Australian researchers attempting to establish guidelines for the World Health Organization did a comprehensive survey of past studies, 116 of them with a combined tally of over 25,000 participants. What they determined was that people sixty-five years and older who performed balance and functional exercises were 24 percent less likely to fall than control subjects. People who did both balance and functional exercises combined with other types of exercise for more than three hours a week had a 42 percent lower risk of falls. That's very significant. We would add that it's not just that people who do balance exercises are less likely to fall, it's also that when they do fall, they're less likely to be injured or need medical care.

If you're not moved by fear of falling—when you're young (and even not so young), the difficulties that come with age can be unimaginable—consider that working on balance will improve your overall movement. Mostly when we think about balance, we think about avoiding some obstacle, righting ourselves if we trip or lose our center of gravity and tumble. But we're also constantly employing our balance skills to move easily through space, and this is particularly true in sports and exercise. Some activities themselves enhance balance—particularly those that depend most on balance, such as cycling, soccer, basketball, skiing, ice skating, surfing, gymnastics, yoga, tai chi, qigong. But a little extra balance work can also improve performance in these activities, as well as help you improve your agility and speed in other activities. Perhaps most important, balance work has been shown to help reduce injuries among both professional and recreational athletes.

HORSING AROUND

When our youngest daughter was a baby, she had a real love affair with her pacifier. She'd go to bed with it, it would inevitably fall out of her mouth while she was sleeping, and then she'd cry because she couldn't find it when she woke up. That meant we had to wake up, too. Our pediatrician had a great solution. "Pepper her crib with twenty pacifiers," he said. "That way there will always be one within reach." Worked like a charm.

We also took the doctor's advice and spun it into a way to practice balance. Scattered around our home and office are all kinds of different balance tools. They're just there so we use them (as do all the visitors to our house). While we're waiting for something to heat up in the microwave or talking on the phone in the living room, we'll practice balancing on a Slack Block, a brick-shaped training implement that's like a slackline (flat webbing strung between two poles for walking on) in miniature. Out in back we have a genuine slackline. One of Kelly's favorite things is to BBQ and slackline.

What having balance tools around allows us to do is just horse around, with a healthy payoff. The great thing about balance training is that it doesn't have to be a formal workout you write into your schedule. Just create little opportunities for you to practice. There are tons of balance tools out there, from BOSU balls and balance boards to mini trampolines. Just play around on them for a few minutes. You could ride a skateboard around your driveway. Play hopscotch with (or without) your kids. One intrepid friend of ours made a balance beam from a PVC pipe.

You don't even need tools. Find something that feels playful. Stand on one leg while you brush your teeth or wash the dishes. Practice yoga tree pose or hop back and forth over an imaginary line while you watch TV. Have a low wall in your backyard? See if you can stay steady as you walk across the wall. Tread barefoot back and forth on textured surfaces to give your feet some input. As a kid you no doubt did all these kinds of things. Now is the time to rediscover what you liked so much about it. (It's fun!)

Physical Practice: Balance Exercises and Mobilizations

Short of being in an athletic program, the only time people seem to do balance work is when something has happened—injury, maybe surgery—and they're working with a fitness trainer or physical therapist. Speaking as professionals, we can tell you there's no reason you need to go to a professional for balance training. You can do a lot of the work just standing at your kitchen counter.

Our physical practice for balance includes a few simple things. The first element is the Y-Balance Mobilization, based on a test that is often given to athletes to assess their balance and risk for injury. It will help you work on dynamic balance—balance while moving. The second element is jumping, preferably with a jump rope, but it doesn't have to be. Rapidly rising up and down on your toes *as if* you're jumping is a form of jumping, and gives you a lot of the same benefits as jumping rope. Since by now you know we're fond of old sayings, here's another one: When you stop jumping, you start dying. Maybe that's a little extreme, but consider that jumping not only keeps your balance systems in shape, it also gets the organs in your viscera cavity moving around, which is beneficial for the health of pretty much all the crucial systems keeping you alive. And there's another bonus, particularly for women, says Stacy Sims, PhD, author of *Next Level: Your Guide to Kicking Ass, Feeling Great, and Crushing Goals Through Menopause and Beyond:* bone building. Sims, an exercise physiologist and nutrition scientist, introduced us to a persuasive study that showed that, in premenopausal women, sixteen weeks of high-impact jump training—jumping ten or twenty times, twice daily, with thirty seconds of rest between each jump—improves hip bone density. If you're not going to do it for your balance, do it for your bones!

The final part of your homework involves ways to sensitize the tissues in your lower legs and feet. It's essentially self-massage. You may be surprised how stiff your lower extremities feel.

Y-Balance Mobilization

To do this move, you'll have to imagine that you are standing in the center of a large Y on the floor. You'll be reaching your foot out in different directions and eyeballing how far your reach extends. You can bend your knee or lean if it helps you to reach. The goal is to reach, breathe for three breaths, and stay balanced.

Stand barefoot on the floor in an open, uncluttered space. Imagine you are standing in the middle of a Y. The single line of the Y goes out in front of you and the two "spears" of the top part of the Y go behind you to your right and to your left. Balancing on one leg, reach the other leg as far forward as you can without losing your balance toward the bottom of the Y and touch your toes to the floor. Hold for three breaths. Next, reach the same foot out to its same side and behind you to touch the top of the Y. Again, reach as far as possible without losing your balance and hold for three breaths. Next, reach the same foot behind your other leg as far

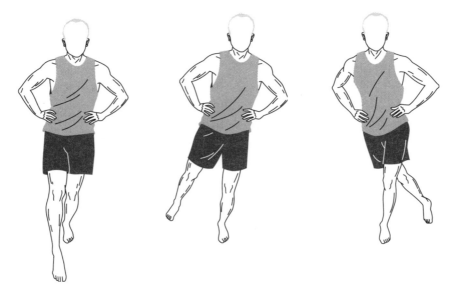

While the Y-Balance Mobilization is formal in its directions,
feel free to play around and discover tricky positions for yourself!

as possible, without losing your balance, to the opposite side to touch the other top of the Y (as if you were bowling). Hold for three breaths. Repeat on the other side.

BALANCE-ENHANCING BOUNCING AND JUMPING

How do we love jumping? Let us count the ways. Besides building balance capabilities, it gets your heart rate up, your blood flowing, and calories burning. For all these reasons, it's an excellent way to warm up for any workout, and by using it as your exercise prep, you'll be killing two birds with one stone—warmup and balance training.

Jumping Rope

Holding a rope in both hands and keeping your torso upright, do 100 to 200 jumps with both feet. Stay on your toes as you jump; you don't need to jump high, just an inch or two off the ground. Next, bend and raise your left leg slightly and jump 50 to 100 times on your right foot. Switch sides.

Or

Bouncing

With your hands resting lightly on a counter or one hand resting on a wall, rise up on your toes and quickly bounce up and down 50 times. You don't need to lower your heels to the ground each time; just drop them partway as you bounce. Next, bend and raise your left leg slightly and bounce 25 times on your right foot. Switch sides.

Bone Saw

This move gets into the tissues in your calf and heel cord. It's the kind of self-massage that might feel a little uncomfortable, but the payoff of decreasing tightness in the area is worth it.

Place a cushion on the floor and get down on your hands and knees, shins atop the cushion. Angle the bottom of your left leg toward the right (shins still atop the cushion) and place the ankle at the bottom of your calf.

Using a sawing motion and applying pressure, move your ankle across the lower calf, working down toward your heel. Saw back up again. Repeat for three to five minutes. Switch sides.

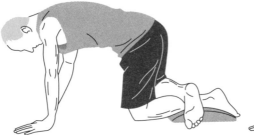

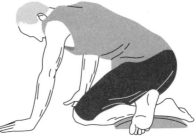

No equipment? No problem. Why is it called the Bone Saw? You will see.

Long sustained pressure can improve how your legs feel.

Calf Stretch Crossover

This might look like a classic calf stretch, but making one small adjustment—stepping your opposite foot across—changes the dynamic. Stepping across puts the hip into extension and also gets deeper into the tissues of the calf.

Stand on top of a curb or a block. Drop your right heel down to the ground so that your foot is angled up. Next, cross your left leg over your right and hold the position for five to ten breaths. Also see if you can't squeeze your glutes on the involved side. Repeat on the other side.

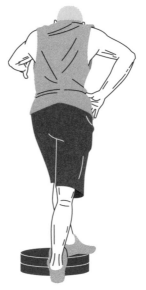

Upgrade the classic with a step "across" and a solid glute squeeze.

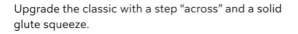

Foot Play

This exercise is exactly what it sounds like.

While sitting on the floor or couch, pull one foot up and massage the heel, arch, ball, and top of the foot. Use your fingers to spread your toes and to twist the front of your foot back and forth. (You've probably seen people wearing toe-spreader shoes. It turns out that your spreaders are already built in—they're called fingers.) Try to wring your feet out, bend and extend your toes. Do this for several minutes, but don't limit yourself. Spend as long as you like on one foot, then switch sides.

Interlacing is a fantastic way to meet your feet again.

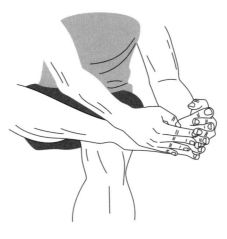

VITAL SIGN **9**

CREATE A MOVEMENT-RICH ENVIRONMENT

ASSESSMENT
Sitting Inventory

PHYSICAL PRACTICE
Setting Up a Standing Workstation; Dynamic Sitting

A FEW YEARS AGO, we heard that a large company with headquarters in the Bay Area had a bright idea. It installed software on employee computers that locked the workers out for five minutes every hour on the hour, a health initiative designed to get workers out of their chairs and moving around. It succeeded. Since they couldn't work, many employees figured they might as well amble around the office or head to the breakroom for a cup of coffee. At the very least they'd get up and stretch. The lockout policy gave their bodies a respite from the L-shaped position demanded by their desk chairs, and it also had the unexpected consequence of fostering employee camaraderie. It helped people become happier at work.

The computer lockout is what we call *creating a movement-rich environment*. It's a way to limit or even take away choices so that you move more. What it's NOT is a strategy dependent on having you give up your desk chair. We're not going to wag a finger at you and tell you to never sit down and look at your computer, or give up your smartphone, or become a Luddite. Today's populace—and our kids—are never going to relinquish technology. Zoom is never going away. Almost everyone in the world now has a personal phone. It's all here to stay, at least until the next technological revolution. So what we need is a different approach, a way to work within our present-day circumstances that honors bodies still built to move as if we were living in prehistoric times.

By design, we're meant to be in motion all day, not necessarily in grand gestures like an hour in the pool or on a running path, but by frequently changing positions, adjusting the body's load, fidgeting. There's always a bit of derisiveness directed at people who "can't sit still," but we'd argue that those people have the right idea. Moving often is imperative whether you're sitting or not.

When addressing Vital Sign 4, we talked about the health consequences of sedentariness, and specifically of sitting too many hours a day. We think you get it by now: Sitting, especially for long periods of time, is not great, and exercise does not cancel out the time you spend in the warm embrace of a chair. Yet that isn't the whole message we want to convey. It's not so much that sitting is bad as it is that moving is better. We actually love sitting. Sitting (especially when you do it on the floor) is awesome. But the truth is, you're way less likely to move while sitting. And sitting shouldn't be your choice for the whole day—which for many people it is. Estimates of how much Americans sit on average vary from six to ten hours a day or, stated another way, from 50 to 70 percent of their waking hours. However, that seems low to us if you think about what a sedentary person's typical day is really like. Eat breakfast and read news (half hour), drive to work (half hour), work at desk till lunch (four hours), eat lunch (one hour), back to desk (three hours), drive home (half hour), eat dinner (half hour), watch TV (two hours)—which amounts to twelve hours, eleven if you subtract some time for minimal to-and-fro walking. There are people who do this for years on end. We know that takes a toll on so many factors, including the body's musculature and other moving parts.

If you are integrating walking into your day à la Vital Sign 4, you are already on your way to moving more and sitting fewer hours. To our mind, the best way to continue working movement into your life is to stand for a greater proportion of your day. Standing is where the action is—that is, people who stand more also tend to move more. While it also has some benefits in and of itself, what we really love about standing is that it's a gateway to movement. Most of those movements may be small, but there's a significant cumulative effect that's well worth chasing.

With that proclamation, you might expect that we'd be asking you to inventory how many hours a day you spend standing. But we're not going to do that. Standing isn't the end-all, be-all. It's just another way—along with walking, along with exercising—to spend time *not sitting*. We want to acknowledge that some people aren't able to stand much (if at all) during a typical day and that there are also plenty of ways to move more within the confines of a chair and/or by taking little movement breaks. But for most of you, lowering the hours you spend sitting is going to be the most movement-positive strategy. So let's see where you're starting from, then we'll talk about ways to get you up and moving for a greater part of the day.

Assessment: Sitting Inventory

It has only been in the last several years, with study after damning study calling it out as a health risk, that prolonged sitting has even entered the general population's radar. And other than a broadly worded recommendation to "limit" sedentary behavior, there are still no official guidelines for exactly how much time we should limit our sitting to. We can, however, look to the research, and what some of the best research says is this (repeating what we noted on pages 101–102): Women and men who sit more than six hours a day are, respectively, 37 percent and 18 percent more likely to die before people who sit less than three hours a day.

Given this data, and given what's practical for most (diligent) people, we believe aiming to curb sitting to six hours a day is a reasonable ask.

Plus, although we're not experts in mortality, we are experts in movement, and we think this number squares with how much sitting the body can stand before it begins to take a toll on mobility. You, too—whether you know it or not—are an expert on movement. How well do you move after hunkering down in a chair for ten to twelve hours? We wager that you feel stiff and clunky, and maybe even experience discomfort. You don't need a study to tell you that a king-size dose of sitting is detrimental to your body.

Still, sitting is so fundamental to modern daily life that many people ignore the damage it does, let alone realize how many hours they actually spend in the same position day after day. If you're one of them, now is your chance to find out. This assessment will take you through a twenty-four-hour period during which you'll note any time you sit in a chair, park yourself on a stool or bench or bed (while sitting, not lying down), or nestle your body into a sofa. We suggest doing the assessment on a typical weekday, weekdays being when most people spend a good share of the day sitting.

There are a few types of sitting that get a pass: sitting or squatting on the floor, or exercising while sitting. Cyclists, rowers, kayakers, and other exercisers who work out in a seated position, you don't need to add that time to your sitting inventory.

PREPARATION

This test is very simple. You'll just need a piece of paper and a pencil to write down the number of hours you sit, plus a little math to add up the hours and minutes. If you'd like help, there are plenty of sitting calculators on the internet (search "sitting calculators") that let you add hours by category (eating breakfast, morning work time, etc.). They then do the math for you.

THE TEST

Beginning from the time you get up in the morning to the time you hop into bed in the evening, track the time you spend sitting. Exceptions: sitting or squatting on the floor; exercising in a seated position.

WHAT YOUR RESULTS MEAN

Your score is the number of hours you spent sitting. Round minutes below 30 down, minutes above 30 up (e.g., 7 hours 26 minutes is 7 hours; 7 hours 45 minutes is 8 hours).

If you're surprised by how much you sit, you're not alone. Some of the most well-trained athletes we know get a shock when they calculate their numbers. What's important now is that you're aware of it and can take steps (literal steps) to avoid prolonged periods of sitting. Here's what your score tells you about where you are and where you need to go.

> **6 hours or less**—We are impressed! Unless you have a job that requires standing (and maybe you do), it's not easy to hit this mark. Keep it up.
>
> **7 to 9 hours**—Depending where you are in this range, we give you a B+ to a C+. If you're at 9 hours, it may seem like a big leap to get down to 6, but our experience tells us that once you start spending more time out of a chair, change will come fairly easily. You'll begin wanting to sit less.
>
> **10 to 12 hours**—You earn a solid C-. You will need to reformat your days somewhat substantially, but we've seen hundreds of people do it. So can you.
>
> **13+ hours**—We regret to say that you are failing in this one area. The most important thing for you to remember, and we'll reiterate this again later, is that you don't have to change overnight. It's not only fine to gradually increase the time you spend on your feet rather than in a chair, it's also preferable.

WHEN SHOULD YOU RETEST?
Daily.

Taking a Stand

In some ways, the physical practice for this Vital Sign might be called Vital Sign 4, Part II. Whereas some of the other physical practices in this book aim to get you to move in specific ways in order to extend your range of motion—the hip extension and shoulder rotation mobilizations are great examples—both Vital Sign 4 and Vital Sign 9 just aim to get you to move more, to be less sedentary. Steps per day is a big part of that, but unless it's part of your job, chances are you can't be walking all day long. That's where standing comes in. If you stand, you're going to end up moving more. It's that simple.

Granted, strictly speaking, standing is *not moving,* and it can be pretty stationary if you allow it to be. But chances are you won't. In our experience, standing makes you *want* to move. In fact, for comfort's sake, it requires that you move. If you watch someone stand for more than a few minutes—or recall any time you yourself have stood for a long time—you might notice how hard it is to stay still. You might sway your hips, shuffle your feet around, bend one knee then the other, shift your weight, find something to lean on, cross and uncross your arms. We've seen people at concerts pull their leg into a yoga tree pose just to deal with the discomfort of standing. Few people—and a nod here to the guards at Buckingham Palace—can stand like a sentry for any length of time; the body will move around to establish stability and equilibrium.

These moves are what you'd call fidgeting. Actually, some researchers prefer the term "spontaneous physical activity" (SPA) to describe what is an unconscious drive for movement without any reward attached to it (in other words, swaying your hips or crossing your arms doesn't help you grab a book off a shelf or get you closer to a bag of Cheetos). Fidgeting/SPA also falls into the category of NEAT—non-exercise activity thermogenesis ("thermogenesis" is another name for calorie burning). Besides fidgeting, NEAT includes things like taking a grocery cart for a spin around the market, getting up from your desk to go to the restroom, typing, and bending down to tie your shoes. And it's NEAT that may be partly responsible for separating the overweight from those who are able to maintain a healthy weight. People who are fidgety and get up and move a lot tend to be thinner.

One of the preeminent researchers in the field of sedentary studies is James Levine, MD, formerly the codirector of the Mayo Clinic/Arizona State University Obesity Solutions Initiative. Levine has helped shine a spotlight on the downside of sitting. ("Excessive sitting," Dr. Levine once told *The New York Times*, "is a lethal activity.") Among the many studies to come out of his lab was one that compared the calorie cost of doing nothing with various activities. The results tell the story:

ENERGY EXPENDITURE AS COMPARED TO LYING STILL:

Sitting motionless—6% ↑

Fidgeting while sitting—54% ↑

Standing motionless—13% ↑

Fidgeting while standing—94% ↑

Walking 1 mph—154% ↑

Walking 2 mph—202% ↑

Walking 3 mph—292% ↑

From our own "lab," Juliet ran some numbers and figured out that by standing for eight hours a day (she has a standing desk), she burned 275 more calories than if she'd been plopped down on a couch or chair for the same amount of time. Over 365 days, that's an additional 100,000 calories a year, or the equivalent of running thirty-eight marathons (the average runner burns about 100 calories per mile). And that's not even counting fidgeting—just calorie expenditure from being erect. Even if she reduced the number of stand-up days to 260 (the average number of business days in a year), that's still 71,000 calories burned—or the equivalent of running twenty-seven marathons. When you're burning calories like that, you have a lot more flexibility about what you can eat.

If you care about calories, that has to be a good incentive to sit less and stand more. But there are other good reasons as well. Researchers in Japan have found that workers who decreased their sitting time also decreased their shoulder and neck pain. Other studies have found that using adjustable sit-stand workstations leads to less back pain. On the flip side, we know that stagnating in a seated position is an invitation to back pain and that back pain makes people move less in their chairs—a vicious cycle if ever there was one.

When you sit for long periods of time and feel pain, it's not hard to connect the two. But there are also plenty of things caused by prolonged sitting that you might not even know are happening until it's too late. Among them: impaired vascular function, high blood pressure, poor blood sugar metabolism, inflammation, reduced blood flow to the brain, and even blunting the beneficial effects of exercise, such as lowering triglycerides and insulin levels. One reason this happens is that when you're seated in a chair, your leg musculature becomes very passive and consequently doesn't require much energy. In response, many things, including blood flow and blood sugar metabolism, slow down. If, on the other hand, you're standing, your legs are loaded—they have to work to support your upper body weight. This taxes the system for the better.

Researchers at the School of Nutrition and Health Promotion at Arizona State University demonstrated this in a study that involved measuring post-meal blood sugar in nine overweight participants under varying conditions. On the first day of the study, the subjects just sat for eight hours. A week later they stood for part of the day. A week after that they cycled for a time, and a week after that they walked. All the interventions were spaced out—the first one was ten minutes long, then they escalated to fifteen-, twenty-, and thirty-minute intervals—adding up to two and a half hours of non-sitting per eight-hour day. Not surprisingly, the walking and cycling intervals prompted the best blood sugar numbers (cycling came in first), but simply standing also significantly improved blood sugar metabolism.

Like anything, standing can be taken to extremes. No one is suggesting you should never sit down, especially as you begin adding in these mobilizations. If you're not used to it and you go from standing about an hour a day to standing twelve hours, you may feel like you've just completed a triathlon: achy. (There's an antidote to that—see pages 205–206.) That said, as cofounders of an organization that installed standing desks in elementary schools (we'll tell you that story in You're Never Too Young to Start: StandUp Kids, page 236) and authors of a book about how to break the sitting habit (*Deskbound: Standing Up to a Sitting World*), we've heard every argument *against* standing and we have a comeback for every single one of them. As noted, Juliet figured out that standing during the day boosted her yearlong calorie burning substantially. Naysayers like to note that when you compare one hour of standing to one hour of sitting the difference in energy expenditure is not big. Perhaps. But we subscribe to the Aggregation of Marginal Gains Theory.

The Aggregation of Marginal Gains is a riff on business principles used with great success by Dave Brailsford, who became head of British Cycling in 2002. Brailsford, an MBA and former competitive cyclist, was handed a team that hadn't won an Olympic gold medal in seventy-six years. Daunted by the challenge ahead of him, Brailsford decided to think small and employ a principle he learned in business school: that compounded improvements could result in significant gains. Applied to cycling, this meant breaking down everything that went into competitive riding and endeavoring to improve each thing by 1 percent. So the team worked on little details like keeping their bike tires clean, bringing their own pillows and mattresses to competitions so they'd get a good night's sleep, and employing proper hand washing and other illness-avoidance tactics. By 2008, the team had won seven out of ten velodrome golds at the Beijing Olympics. They then repeated their winning performance four years later in London.

So, if you tell us that there's not a huge calorie jump when you jump up from your chair, our reply is, So what? Because with *consistency* we've not only seen those small numbers compound, we've also seen other benefits amass over time. To reiterate, when you stand, you're likely to fidget, so any calorie chart that says standing only burns ten or so more calories than sitting isn't telling the whole story: Fidgeting ups the energy expenditure numbers. Plus, added to the mix are the stiffness-countering benefits of fidgeting while standing and the fact that standing takes you out of the dreaded C shape we talked about in Vital Sign 5. Standing also just naturally leads to more steps. When we get phone calls and are already standing, we're more likely to pace as we talk than if we had to get up from the chair. It's easier to walk over to a colleague's desk rather than email because you're already up—no having to drag yourself out of the chair. Sitting is anesthetizing; standing is invigorating, which is also going to make you less prone to that 3 p.m. afternoon slump.

There's a particular gain for exercisers as well. Too often people who work out in the morning or during lunch go right from redlining their internal RPMs to sitting flaccidly in a chair. We know that is not the best way to facilitate maximal adaptation to exercise, nor does it give the heart rate and temperature time to slowly return to normal. Also, encased in a chair (or a car's seat), you're not promoting circulation, which can cause your muscles and connective tissue to stiffen up. That's why swimmers like Michael Phelps move over to the warm-down pool after a race, and why horses are walked around the track after the Kentucky Derby has been run. One of the nice things about setting yourself up with a movement-rich environment is that you don't have to cool down. Say you're working at home and you've just gotten off your Peloton bike. You can go right to your stand-up desk, and the fidgeting and changing of positions you'll inevitably do will help you cool down.

On the flip side, what do you think the difference will be between going for a run after standing at a desk for three hours and going out for a run after sitting for three hours? You're going to have a different experience. You can test this. Sit for an hour and go sprint; then stand and fidget for an hour and go sprint. Your time post-standing is going to best your post-sitting time.

YOU'RE NEVER TOO YOUNG TO START: STANDUPKIDS

It began with, of all things, a sack race. In 2013, we volunteered at our daughters' elementary school field day, helping the kids get into the sacks for the race across the yard. We were astonished at how many kids, some as young as six, didn't have the range of motion to easily get into the sack, let alone the fitness ability to hop through the entire race. Many of the kids were overweight, too.

Most parents probably wouldn't have thought much of it, but you know us and movement: We were galvanized. Sitting—because that was clearly what most kids were doing for a ridiculous number of hours per day—was harming kids, and we wanted to do something about it. A year after that fateful sack race, Juliet founded StandUp Kids and began building a nonprofit educational group intended to change how much children were sitting during the day.

The next step was to take tangible action. Together, we went into our oldest daughter's fourth-grade classroom and converted it to the first-known all standing/moving classroom in California. A few months later we funded a standing conversion for the rest of the fourth grade and for one first-grade class, for a total of a hundred kids at standing desks. With fundraising ($110K!), we were able to convert the whole 450 desks in the school to stand-ups by 2015. The following year we learned that over 27,000 kids nationwide had access to a standing desk during the day. In 2017, StandUp Kids was able to provide a $50,000 grant for standing desks in public schools.

What we found was that the kids took to the standing desks immediately. The only ones who complained a little were the fifth graders, which was understandable—they had been doing the most sitting of all the students. But after two weeks every kid, even the fifth graders, had adapted. Occasionally we'd get pushback from a parent. "My son is so tired when he gets home." And that's a bad thing? We want kids' days to tire them out. That way they sleep well, which gives them the rest they need to grow properly. And the payoff for kids spending four hours a day standing and moving rather than sitting is priceless.

Mark Benden, PhD, professor at the Texas A&M Health Science Center, School of Public Health, has been studying the effects of standing desks on children for some years. Benden's research has shown that above and beyond the extra calorie expenditure (17 percent more than seated students, almost double that for overweight kids), standing students were more focused and less disruptive.

Many a parent and grandparent has asked why kids need to stand in school; after all, they never did. But for many parents that's because they 1) didn't have the same level of technology we do today, and 2) didn't get driven to school. In 1969, 48 percent of five- to fourteen-year-olds walked or biked to school. In 2009, 13 percent walked or biked. In 2014, 10 percent did. With many kids now schooling at home, the number today may be even lower.

Obviously, converting to a standing desk is only one way to keep kids healthy, but it's relatively easy to get kids to be enthusiastic about it. Most like it a lot more than broccoli!

The Change "Up"

Our ultimate goal is to have you spend less time sitting in the same position. There are lots of ways to do that, whether it be by using a standing desk or toggling back and forth between a standing and a sitting desk, taking frequent breaks from your regular sitting desk, doing some of your working/viewing at a kitchen counter, or making a personal policy of not sitting on public transportation or in waiting rooms. You can do any or all of the above, changing your strategies as the day allows. You can even stay seated and employ some of the movement tactics we recommend (page 244). We want to meet you where you are, but we also hope you'll shoot for the moon: sitting only six or fewer hours a day.

As sedentary as we are as a society, there is undoubtedly something in the zeitgeist telling us to get up out of our chairs. As you may have noticed, there are now phone apps, computer prompts, smartwatches, fitness trackers, and other devices that encourage you to stand up at various times. Employers are also thinking of creative ways to get their employees to stand up and move around. Our friend Jim implemented a very clever policy at his company (and it wasn't a suggestion—it was a policy) called Walk/Talk/Click. The deal was, if you needed to communicate with a colleague, the first thing you had to do was walk to the person's desk to see if you could talk to them in person. If they were busy on a call or in the middle of something, they'd flip on the little light Jim had installed in everyone's cubicle. If your attempt at face-to-face communication failed, you could then call the person. If you couldn't reach them that way, you could finally resort to email (*click*). Jim was trying to foster better face-to-face communication, but also wanted to get his employees to move—and they really had to, because the office space was large, with multiple stories.

Occasionally we'll hear some grumbling about how productivity and thought are disrupted by tactics like Jim's policy or by devices' *dings* and *beeps* reminding people to stand. Yet as some research suggests, that standing can actually enhance productivity. In 2016, researchers at Texas A&M Health Science Center, School of Public Health, published a study that looked at productivity in call center workers provided with sit-stand desks over the course of six months. Half of the 167 participants were provided with the adjustable desks while half had regular desks and desk chairs. The standers—who ended up sitting 1.6 hours less per day than their counterparts—showed themselves to be increasingly more productive than the sitters (based on the success of their calls), beginning at 23 percent more productivity the first month and 53 percent more productivity at six months. The standers also reported less body discomfort. The call center standers' productivity squares with what we know about kids who use stand-up desks: Standing is associated with significant improvements in executive function and working-memory capabilities in students.

Employer-led programs, devices that promote less sitting—they are all good. But when it comes down to brass tacks, you are going to be the one responsible for opting out of the easy chair. There will always be desk chairs, subway seats, waiting room benches, and living room couches beckoning to you, and it's human nature to want to avail yourself of their comfort. But what we've seen is that when you change your mindset about sitting, it gradually becomes less attractive. "No, I'll stand" becomes not a nicety when someone offers you a seat on the bus, but something you actually want to do because it feels good. You'll find, too, that there are choices you can make that you may have never noticed before. For instance, when we go to a big conference, instead of finding a seat in the front or middle rows, we stand behind the very last one. Usually no one sits in the last row, so if it's a long presentation, we can stand as long as feels right, then slip into a seat when we're ready. In the same vein, there's no law that says you have to sit at a table to pack groceries when you're volunteering at a food bank or that you have to take a seat in the examination room while the vet is examining your pet. No reason you can't stand while you wait for your take-out food. Or stand up and move around instead of sitting with a cup of coffee to avoid the afternoon slump. Once you've got a "sit less" mentality, all kinds of opportunities will present themselves.

For many people, the biggest obstacle to standing is their desk. We're big advocates of desks that allow you stand, but there are a few misconceptions around them that drive us crazy. The first is that you need to spend a lot of money on a standing or adjustable sit-stand desk. You *could*—and if you want to spend a few thousand for the Ferrari of standing desks, knock yourself out. You can even get a treadmill desk if you're really committed to moving. But don't let the perfect, bright-and-shiny technology be the enemy of good. There are plenty of effective, inexpensive options, including raisable platforms that fit on top of a regular desk and can also be used on the floor if you'd like to do your work or gaming or viewing or whatever sitting cross-legged (an idea that you know from Vital Sign 1 we support). There are also no-cost options, like taping a few cardboard boxes together, placing them on the desk you already have, and sticking your computer on top. *Voilà*. You have a stand-up desk. Do you have a high kitchen counter? If you have some coffee-table books you can use to elevate your laptop, you, too, are in possession of a standing desk. Be creative. When we first began recommending standing desks to professional and recreational athletes, we received photographs of desk hacks from all over the world. A particular favorite was the one built from a pile of bricks, with a tower on one side to hold a computer monitor and a board perched on lower-level bricks to hold the keyboard. Genius!

The other pet peeve we have about the standing desk issue is a not-uncommon complaint: "My employer won't provide me with one." But your employer is not in charge of your health; you are. If you want a standing desk, make one or get a raisable platform for your office desk. Don't wait for a note from your doctor or for your bosses to discover their largesse—though we can think of at least one way you can nudge them forward. A friend was working at a company that said they'd buy him a standing desk, but they were dragging their feet. So he grabbed the ugliest, dirtiest cardboard box he could find, brought it to the office, slapped it down on his desk, and went to work on his now raised computer. He had a brand-new standing desk by the end of the next week.

Physical Practice: Setting Up a Standing Workstation; Dynamic Sitting

We created the sitting inventory and its scoring to highlight what research indicates promotes both good musculoskeletal and overall health. The ideal is six hours or less of sitting per day, but you can also think about it another way: *Mix* sitting and standing throughout your day. It doesn't have to be an either-or thing. Do it in chunks: Sit for twenty, stand for ten. Fidget, change positions. In other words, *move!* When you're standing straight ahead, try to keep your feet in the reference foot position (page 120), but don't worry about it too much, because most of the time you'll be moving this way and that.

The important thing is to give yourself choices. You're not going to stand and work if you don't have a place to stand and work, so get busy figuring out how to install any of the standing workstations we mentioned earlier. Once you've got the equipment, we've got guidelines for using it safely and efficiently. When you're not standing (and if you're not going to be standing at all), we still want you moving. Part of this physical practice is learning how to be less sedentary in your chair.

One final note before you get going. If you're walking and engaging in the mobilizations in this book, your body is going to be more durable and better able to handle longer periods of sitting. All the better if you exercise, too. In other words, you have more flexibility. Maybe you don't have to hit six hours or less of sitting; maybe you can sit somewhat longer without repercussions. As always, listen to your body. By the same token, if you're absolutely not going to use a standing workstation, you may have to really double your efforts to move within the space you're in. Take the Dynamic Sitting section to heart.

SETTING UP A STANDING WORKSTATION

Whichever kind of standing desk you choose, top-of-the-line or home-made Rube Goldberg contraption, there are some setup fundamentals that will make it tenable for movement, efficiency, and comfort. Here are five things you need to know about setting up a standing workstation, starting from the bottom up.

1 GROUND CONTROL If the surface beneath your workstation is very hard, you'll end up moving more to chase comfort. That might sound like a good thing, but it may also be an indication that your feet will suffer from the rigidity of the floor beneath them. See how it feels. If after a few days you feel pain, either wear a more cushioned shoe or add cushioning in the form of a throw rug or exercise mat. There are also many antifatigue mats on the market created especially for people who stand for long periods of time. Standing static without movement options on a hard surface is a fast track to uncomfortable.

2 DESK HEIGHT Many fixed-height standing desks come in at 40 to 42 inches. Then there are adjustable solutions that sit on top of the desk you already have and the desks you make yourself, which give you more leeway in terms of surface height. To state the obvious, everyone's body is different, so don't go by a particular measurement. Instead, use this rule of thumb: Stand as instructed in the proper standing position (see number 4). Bend your arms so that your forearms are parallel to the floor. Your desk should be at elbow height, plus one inch (to allow for keyboard height). We say *should*, not must, because you've got to see how it feels. If it doesn't feel good, that's a sign you need to adjust it either up (this is where books come in handy) or down. If you're contemplating a fixed-height desk, be cautious before you buy. You can always build it up by placing your keyboard on books, but you can't scale it back down.

3 POSITIONING AIDS We contend that a workstation is not a workstation unless it has accoutrements that give you positioning options. Bartenders figured out long ago that if you want people to hang around and spend more money, you need a counter at a height they can lean on and a place they can put a foot up to take some of the load off their lumbar spine. That's why every pub has a rail at the base of the bar. Taking a page from the bartender playbook will increase the comfort of standing by helping you move into different shapes and, in doing so, keep you on your feet longer. Placing a barstool—preferably one with a flat seat and squared edges that's about the height of your inseam—behind you will give you a surface to occasionally lean back against, perch on (perching is way better than sitting, since you still need to work a bit to keep your balance), or rest your foot on. When you lean back or perch, it should look a little like standing and a little like sitting. The other workstation essential we recommend is a foot support that, by allowing you to prop up one foot like on a bar rail, will make it easier to stand comfortably. You can use the lower rails on your stool or the seat of a chair to raise a foot (or, in the case of a chair seat, rest a knee), or place a box or slant board underneath your desk. A swinging footrest, called a "fidget bar," is another under-desk option. You'll find that if you have the right accessories next to you, your body will naturally figure out how to use them to lighten its load and stay in equilibrium.

4 PROPER STANDING POSITION   The point of using a standing desk is to move more, so you're going to automatically assume many different positions during your standing sessions. But during those times when you're standing straight, the best position is the reference foot position (see page 120). To refresh your memory: As you are standing comfortably with your feet straight and underneath your hips, you should have 50 percent of your weight on the balls of your feet and 50 percent of your weight on the heels. Also, if you look down, your ankles should be in the middle of your feet, not collapsing in, out, toward the front, or toward the back. If your ankles lean one way or the other or your knees knock in, you're not in a great position.

5 YOU'RE OFF TO THE RACES   When we say you're off to the races, we really mean it: You need to train for using a standing workstation like you'd train for a marathon. Just as you wouldn't go from spending your waking days on the couch to running 26 miles, you shouldn't go for twenty years of sitting to standing eight hours a day. If you do, it's going to be painful. A lot of overeager people who think they've found the key to good health end up pushing the button to lower their standing desk and never raise it again. So take it slow. Start out with a half hour a day and increase at a pace that feels right.

DYNAMIC SITTING

We understand that some people won't or can't use a standing workstation. We also acknowledge that when most people sit, except for the tiny pecking of their fingers, they are essentially motionless. Don't let that be your MO. Moving more while seated can be done! But don't take our word for it. James Levine's lab, in a 2016 study, showed that using a chair or footrest designed to promote fidgeting increased energy expenditure by 20 percent. So, whether you sit all the time or rotate between sitting and standing, here are some ways to keep moving.

BREATHE

This isn't so much about moving as it is about avoiding the tendency to curl up like a shrimp while sitting at a desk, straining your neck, your shoulders, your back, and on down the line. When seated, ensure that your body is well organized by getting into a shape where you can take a deep breath. If you can't take a deep breath, it's a sign that you're not in a very movement-friendly position. Once you're where you can breathe fully, then you can think about starting to move more.

GEAR UP

A few years ago, we were asked for advice on setting up an office for an author who'd already written two bestselling memoirs and was about to start on his third. A standing desk was out of the question; he needed to sit to focus. But he was also aware that sitting for all the hours he'd need to write the book would be hard on his body. In fact, he'd already been doing a lot of sitting and it was taking a toll on his golf game. We recommended two things to help the author move more while sitting. One was a fidget bar. There are several of these footrest devices on the market that provide a little resistance as you swing them or push against them (as noted earlier, you can use them with standing desks, too). The other movement-facilitating gear we recommended was a chair that allowed for greater movement of the torso. There exists a whole new seating category called "active seating," which includes chairs, stools, and balls that enable mobility while sitting. We don't have a favorite, just an overall rule of thumb: Your desk chair should not be a cozy little alcove for you to slump into.

RISE UP

Baseball has the seventh-inning stretch. You have the half-hour stretch. Do whatever it takes to remind you to get out of your chair every thirty minutes—an electronic alert on your computer, an alarm on your watch—and OBEY it. Get up for a minute or more and move, whether to stretch, walk to the bathroom or breakroom, or take a lap around your workplace. If you can't stand up, use that half-hour alert to just move more within the confines of your chair.

TAKE MOBILIZATION BREAKS

There are some easy mobility exercises you can do right next to your desk that will help balance out the effects of sitting. The Kneeling Isometric (page 97) helps relieve compression on the spine and promotes good hip extension. You can also do a variation of Elevated Pigeon (page 48) while seated: While sitting in a chair, keeping one foot flat on the floor, bend your other leg and place your ankle on top of your bent knee so that your legs form a 4 shape. Place your hands on your bent leg, lean forward slightly, and rotate toward your left side, then rotate toward your right side. Continue alternating between the two positions for two minutes or as long as possible. Switch sides.

UNLEASH YOUR SUPERPOWER: SLEEP

ASSESSMENT
Hours Count

PHYSICAL PRACTICE
A Better Shut-Eye Plan

Y OU HAVE REACHED the last Vital Sign and it is by no means the least. We wouldn't go as far as to say that without adequate sleep, every other physical practice in this book is moot. However, sleep really is the linchpin, the hub that everything else revolves around. Aside from the innumerable ways that sufficient sleep sustains the body, from cardiovascular health and cognitive function to how we experience pain, it also gives you the energy to follow all the recommendations we've provided thus far. If you're sleeping well, you'll not only be more apt to perform the nine other Vital Sign physical practices, you'll get more out of them, too.

Sleep is the body's time to recuperate from stress and consolidate new information in the brain. It is also critical to overall wellness: Seven out of the fifteen leading causes of death have been linked to deficient sleep. It's for all those reasons that your body tries so hard to warn you that you need more time under the covers. Think about how you feel when you're tired. Slow, unmotivated, enervated. It can color everything you do, including decisions you make pertaining to your body's well-being and mobility. When you're exhausted, you'll be more liable to make unhealthy food choices and sit slumped at your desk.

Granted, this might not happen to you every time you burn the candle at both ends. The human body is incredibly tolerant. We can cram it into awkward positions, eat poorly, sleep hardly at all, and it will still function. Thank goodness for that, because if you're sick, or have a baby, or are immersed in an all-encompassing work project, there will be times when you'd be in real trouble if the human body weren't so forgiving. But tolerating suboptimal living and thriving are two different things. Likewise, skimping on the important things in the short term is poles apart from doing so over weeks, months, or years. You may not experience the damage being done today until somewhere down the line.

According to the Sleep Foundation, 35 percent of people sleep less than seven hours a night. Most of these people probably wish they could sleep more, though—regrettably—for some people, sleeping very little is a point of pride. Business publications love to laud the brilliant CEOs and politicians who supposedly run in high gear on only four hours of sleep a night. Bill Clinton, a famous nonsleeper—until he had a quadruple bypass operation (coincidence or just a lot of stress and unfortunate DNA? probably all of the above)—was told by one of his college professors that great men require less rest than ordinary people. Perhaps there is a small subset of men and women—researchers call them the "sleepless elite"—who by virtue of genetics can do well on less than five hours of sleep per night. But sleep experts say that the sleepless elite number less than 1 percent of the population. No offense, but odds are you're not one of them. We know *we're* not among them. Virtually nobody *doesn't* need seven to nine hours of sleep. Before you go into work and humblebrag, "I got four hours of sleep last night," consider the likely thought bubble in your coworkers', maybe even your boss's, head: "Wow, you're going to be the least efficient worker today, contribute nothing, and make our company worse!"

Although no one would say the COVID-19 pandemic was a good

thing, one by-product of the shift in the way people work has been that many of them are getting more sleep. How that will ultimately play out is unknown right now, but pre-pandemic it was clear that lack of sleep was a global problem. The Centers for Disease Control and Prevention has called sleeplessness a public health problem.

As you might have gathered by now, we're passionate on the subject of sleep, a mindset we hope to pass on to you by sharing all the reasons it should be a priority, as well as some ideas on how to slow to a stop so you get the shut-eye you need. We all know how to go, go, go; not many of us know a healthy way to bring the day to a close. Balance is missing. Better that we take a page from the dirt bike racers' playbook: Ride with the throttle wide open, then slam on the brakes. A few simple sleep strategies can help with that.

So let's see where you're at. Our assessment will help you take an honest look at how many hours of sleep you're accruing on an average night.

Assessment: Hours Count

Whenever we're working with individuals or groups, no matter their stature—professional athletes, military elite, recreational athletes, people who don't exercise at all—we ask them how much sleep they're getting. Then, because people notoriously under- or overreport how much time they spend sleeping, we ask them to count the hours. That's what we're asking you to do now. Take an honest look at how much you're sleeping. Not how much time you spend in bed, but how much time you're actually snoozing. Equally important is how you feel the next day. Sleeping an average of eight hours is great, but the quality of your sleep is critical, too.

Our assessment has limits. A medically led sleep study done at a clinic or hospital can tell you not only if you're getting adequate amounts of sleep but can clock whether you're experiencing the different stages of sleep (more about this later) and help you determine if you have any sleep disorders. Likewise, you can get some idea of sleep stages and night disruptions with a wearable sleep tracker device. There are many to choose among—Garmin, Apple, Oura, and Fitbit are just some of the companies that make them. There are even nonwearable sleep trackers that go on your bed, like the Sleepme+, which monitor all the factors that provide a good night's sleep and adjust the temperature of your mattress to promote deep REM sleep duration. All these devices, both wearable and nonwearable, typically track movement and/or heart rate to give you a morning update on your sleep duration and quality. This can really be useful. We're all for getting more information; sleep trackers are great. But we also believe just calculating your hours of sleep and asking yourself how you feel the next day can be truly eye-opening. Get your slumber number and let's go from there.

PREPARATION

You'll be averaging the number of hours you sleep on three nights. We recommend including a Friday or Saturday night so you can also take a look at whether you're significantly varying your sleep hours between weekdays and weekends. No tools are needed other than a bed and a piece of paper or other place to do the math. You might want to have a notepad on your nightstand so that if you find yourself lying awake you can write down an estimate of how long you were up. Better than leaving it until the morning, when you might forget.

THE TEST

It's simple: Turn out the light and go to bed. The next morning, calculate how long you slept, subtracting any time you woke up during the night, whether to use the bathroom or just lying awake. Try, too, to estimate how long it took you to fall asleep and subtract that time. This may not be perfect, but it will give you a good estimate. (Of course, if you have a sleep tracker, use it.) Complete this process on three average nights, one of them a weekend night or other night where you don't have work the next day. Let's leave naps out of the calculation—we'll talk about them later.

After each night's sleep, also evaluate how your day goes energy-wise. Did you feel sleepy before noon? Did you need caffeine to help you wake up in the morning?

WHAT YOUR RESULTS MEAN

Add up the hours you slept each night and divide by 3. That number is your score.

If you are getting less than seven hours of sleep a night, you are not getting enough. We'd love to pat you on the back and say, "Well, at least you're getting *some* sleep," but that's not what we're going for here. We believe the world would be a healthier and kinder place if we all slept the appropriate amount of time. Don't settle for less! If you are getting seven hours of sleep and find you are still sleepy by 10 or 11 a.m.—a condition that can only be alleviated by caffeine—then consider that maybe you're one of those people who actually need eight or nine hours. If you're hitting those higher numbers and still feeling tired, it's a good idea to talk to your doctor.

WHEN SHOULD YOU RETEST?

Every night! You're (presumably) already going to bed each night, so keep a log of how much you're sleeping.

Vitamin Sleep

When we're tired, most of us hold it together. But if you look at how kids behave when they haven't gotten enough sleep, you get a little window into what the body really thinks about being sleep deprived. When our daughters were young, we prioritized good sleep, making sure that they had consistent bedtimes and naps. We were *those* kinds of parents, and it paid off. As toddlers, the girls would always elicit remarks like, "Your kids are so well behaved. They're such nice kids." We'd always look at each other and laugh, because we were probably getting an F in every other part of parenting, but because our kids were well rested, they were also less prone to emotional highs and lows.

When kids are under two years old, all bets are off. But as they get older and they're falling down on the floor and tantruming, crying, and arguing, it's usually because they're tired. As adults, we don't have the luxury to do the same, although when we're beat, most of us would probably like to beat our fists on the ground as well. If this is how you feel on a daily basis, it's a message from your brain telling you you're doing your body wrong.

Sleep—enough sleep, high-quality sleep—is so vital that we could write a whole book about it. (As many others have—most notably Matthew Walker, PhD, a professor of neuroscience and psychology at UC Berkeley and the director of its Center for Human Sleep Science, whose book *Why We Sleep* has informed a lot of our views.) But if we summarize, you'll get the gist of why we've made it Vital Sign 10.

Your brain is arguably the most important part of your body—without it, nothing else happens. So the fact that the brain depends on sleep to do its job is the most pressing reason to make it a priority. While you're sleeping tonight, your brain will be shuffling things around to make room for the new information you'll be presented with tomorrow. Sleep also allows the brain to create memories and enhances learning, whether it's intellectual fuel you're trying to digest or motor skills you want to improve.

One of the most interesting sleep studies Matthew Walker has done involved asking right-handed participants to learn a left-hand typing sequence. They practiced this motor skill for a while, then were tested on it twelve hours later. Half of the participants had practiced in the evening and had an eight-hour night's sleep before their test. The other half, who'd practiced in the morning, were tested in the evening, no sleep in between. Guess who did better on the test? Those who'd had a full night's sleep. When the other group was tested again after they, too, had slept on it, they showed similar improvement. Walker's assessment: Practice—and sleep—make perfect.

This is one reason it's a well-established fact that athletes perform better when they've adequately satisfied their bodies' demand for sleep. Better reaction time is another. Well-rested athletes also have lower rates of injuries. This is pertinent information for everyone. If you're going to throw the ball with your kid or jump on your bike, you want all things in their best working order. Even if the extent of your athleticism only extends to cleaning the house and maybe a little yard work, you have a body that needs to move, and it will move better with a good night's sleep.

There is more to this than just the brain's role in movement. As you slumber, the body also turns over the cells in your movement-related tissues, repairing muscle and stimulating its growth. With less sleep, less robust musculature. Sleep deprivation can also make you less sensitive to insulin, which can in turn make your tissues more likely to become inflamed and therefore less tolerant to exertion.

How much pain you feel from any musculoskeletal issues you're dealing with can also be influenced by your sleep habits. With sleep deprivation, two things can happen. One is that the part of the brain that telegraphs pain to your consciousness becomes more sensitive. At the same time, the areas that dull the perception of pain—kind of like your body's own inner aspirin—become less active. On the flip and more positive side, if your back is aching on Monday, a good night's sleep may help it hurt less on Tuesday. When people come to us with pain, the first thing we ask them is how much they're sleeping. Sleep is the first line of defense against pain.

If we zoom out and look at the big picture, we see that sleep is also key to overall well-being. In the day-to-day, sleep helps keep the immune system strong, protecting you from viruses like the common cold. In 2015, a team led by a University of California, San Francisco, researcher found that simply sleeping less than six hours a night ups your chance of catching a cold fourfold, no matter your age. Among the interesting studies coming out of the COVID-19 pandemic was one from Beijing that found the less people slept in the week before contracting the virus, the more severe their symptoms. (The study also found that two ends of the activity spectrum—sedentariness and overexertion—increased susceptibility to the disease.)

Even more sobering, a large body of research has also linked sleep deprivation to lowered life expectancy as well as many life-threatening conditions, including diabetes, obesity, depression, heart attack, and stroke. In sleep lab settings, researchers have been able to observe why lack of sleep may trigger some of these maladies. For instance, subject to what amounts to a half night's sleep (four hours), people have increased cortisol release (the fight-or-flight hormone), decreased sensitivity to insulin, and more inflammation, all of which contribute to the type of raised blood glucose levels associated with diabetes. The heart is also placed at risk by lack of sleep. Sleep provides a time for the heart to rest, as evidenced by the slowing of your heart rate as you doze. Blood pressure also drops during sleep. When you don't get the requisite forty winks, the cardiovascular system keeps on working at warp speed, without the time it needs to recover.

One of the ways sleep intersects with Vital Sign 6—Eat Like You're Going to Live Forever—is by affecting appetite. It is well established that lack of sleep is associated with both weight gain and poor food choices, and researchers have begun to tease out why. There is, for one thing, the fact that the more hours you're up, the more likely you are to get hungry and eat. In studies, sleep-deprived subjects often eat more at night than their well-rested counterparts. They also simply consume more calories overall: about 204 more calories a day, according to a 2021 meta-analysis of fifty-four sleep studies. This might not sound like much, but multiply it over weeks and months, and that's a lot of extra calories.

There's some biochemistry at work here. As part of a fifteen-year sleep study in Wisconsin, researchers found that short sleepers (five hours a night) had different levels of appetite-related hormones than long sleepers (eight hours a night). The short sleepers had lower amounts of leptin, which suppresses appetite, and higher levels of ghrelin, which stimulates appetite. Another study looked at sleep's effect on the body's endocannabinoids (eCBs), which are exactly what they sound like—neurotransmitters that have properties similar to those in cannabis, including influencing appetite. University of Chicago researchers measured the levels of eCBs and food intake in men and women after they'd had 8.5 hours of sleep and

4.5 hours of sleep. Each sleep "dose" was for four consecutive days. The short doses of sleep shifted the natural rise-and-fall rhythm of the eCBs, which may explain why, when subjected to reduced shut-eye, the study subjects ate more highly palatable snacks (science-speak for junk food). The researchers reported that people had a harder time resisting snacks when they were sleepy.

"I'VE TRIED EVERYTHING": WHEN YOU STILL CAN'T SLEEP

Insomnia is rampant. Between 10 and 30 percent of adults struggle with chronic insomnia, and the number goes up to 48 percent in older adults. This amounts to a health crisis. Insomnia isn't our area of expertise, so if you're really going sleepless, we urge you to get a sleep study to see what might be going on. But we do have some advice on some things that might help before you get to the point of seeking out a sleep specialist.

First, take a look at the Vital Sign 10 physical practice, go down the list, and employ *every* strategy. We've talked to a lot of people struggling with insomnia who think they've tried everything, only to realize that they really haven't. So consider all the variables: movement, light, sound, technology, routine. Really do try everything, especially the winding-down factor. A short mobility practice before bed can really help downregulate the body and prepare it for sleep.

Also look at what you're ingesting. Alcohol worsens sleep disturbances (as we note on page 262). And the caffeine to wake up, Ambien to go to sleep rotation we see so many people adopting may net you some quantity of sleep and make you feel like you have a semblance of alertness during the day, but sleeping pill–induced sleep is not high-quality sleep, the kind that helps cement learning and memories in the brain. Eventually, this cycle of self-medicating will prove useless and won't likely solve your insomnia problem.

"Insomnia" is a word we toss around anytime we have trouble sleeping, but it's actually a medical disorder. Sometimes what you might be experiencing is just a rough patch. If you're going through a deeply stressful period, which we all do, sleep can be impacted. There's illness and death and divorce and work pressures and family stress. You name it. And it is what it is. Sometimes you just have to weather the storm, then get back to good sleep habits when you can.

Consider, too, that how you handle sleep problems can make a difference. For twenty years, one of the doctors Kelly worked with early in his career struggled to sleep through the night. He'd wake up after four hours and lie there for two hours more, cursing his bad luck and worrying about all the sleep he was losing. Finally, he decided to embrace it. He'd get up, leave his bedroom, read by a low light until he felt sleepy again, then go back to bed and sleep another couple of hours. He found it transformative. Lying awake ruminating about lying awake didn't help; distracting himself from his anxiety with a book did. Was it perfect? No. But whatever can take your mind off insomnia—be it a book on tape, some slow music, a meditation app, counting sheep (really!)—may help. We're fans, too, of Brain.fm, a science-y app that offers music keyed to induce various moods and feelings, including the desire for sleep.

The Body's Braking System

When you're completely exhausted, so tired you can barely keep your eyes open, then finally fall into bed and are dead to the world, sleep seems like the simplest thing in the world. But our body's system for slowing to what's tantamount to a stop is not simple; there's a lot going on leading up to and during those hours you're getting in your forty winks. (Or not getting in your forty winks—on insomnia, see "I've Tried Everything": When You Still Can't Sleep, page 254.)

The need to sleep is generated by a confluence of biological factors. One is the circadian rhythm, the body's internal, approximately twenty-four-hour clock, which largely takes its cues from things in the environment, like light. This inner alarm triggers other physiological mechanisms that help you wake in the morning and make you sleepy as the day winds down. As humans, we pretty much have similar circadian rhythms, but they're not all exactly alike, which explains why you might like to stay up past midnight and your best friend is more of an early to bed, early to rise sort of person. Neither inclination is necessarily better than the other. What matters most is that you get the hours of sleep you need, not when you get them.

The other major catalyst for sleep is known as the "homeostatic sleep-wake drive." Working in conjunction with the circadian rhythm (and as its name suggests), this is what propels you to go to sleep and then to wake hours later. The sleepiness side of this equation—sleep pressure—is triggered by the chemical adenosine, which simultaneously quiets the wakefulness areas of the nervous system while rousing the sleepiness areas. This is noteworthy if you're a physiology geek, but even more so if you're a caffeine freak: Caffeine works by attaching to the receptors that normally host adenosine, blocking the chemical from making you feel sleepy.

While caffeine is beloved for keeping us bright-eyed, melatonin is a supplement prized, sometimes erroneously, for helping us go in the other direction. Melatonin, the kind your body makes itself, is a hormone that begins rising in the bloodstream with the onset of darkness and descends as the sky begins turning light. In this way it helps regulate the circadian rhythm, but melatonin doesn't have a tranquilizing effect—and neither do over-the-counter versions of melatonin, even though many people expect them to. Which isn't to say melatonin can't be helpful: It has been found to help with jet lag and sleep disorders caused by a shift in the sleep-wake cycle.

When things are going well and you stay fast asleep for a good eight hours (or thereabouts), your body will rotate through four sequential sleep stages, each of which has its own role to play in making you a high-functioning human being. The first three stages are known as "non-rapid eye movement" (NREM) sleep. During the first two of these stages, you sleep lightly as your body and brain begin to relax. Muscles untense, breathing and heart rate slow. By the time you hit stage three, deep sleep, you're well into recovery from the day's demands. Your muscles are repairing and growing, and the brain is making room for new memories and data. The real brain work, though, happens during rapid eye movement (REM) sleep, stage four. This is when the brain is active, producing our most vivid dreams, creating memories, and consolidating information we've gleaned throughout the day.

Throughout the night, the body toggles back and forth between NREM and REM sleep. Both are critical, which is why it's so important to get a full seven to nine hours of sleep. Short sleepers can lose substantial amounts of either type of sleep—or both—missing out on their benefits. More alarmingly, deficient REM sleep has been associated with higher death rates in older and middle-aged people. Although the reasons are unknown, research has shown that every 5 percent reduction in REM sleep increases mortality 13 to 17 percent.

It's data like this that has made us very protective, even a little obsessive, about our own sleep. It's not that we've achieved perfection. We can both be prone to sleep disturbances—Kelly because, even if the bedroom is in total darkness and he's wearing an eye mask, he can still perceive when one of our girls has left a light on somewhere in the house, and Juliet because she's susceptible to anxiety-provoked wake-ups. But it's fairly normal to wake during the night, and it becomes even more so as you get older because of age-related changes to the circadian rhythm and hormone production. (The hard part is getting back to sleep—see page 254.)

You may not even be aware of how much you're waking in the night, something that can make you wonder why you're not feeling refreshed in the morning. A few years ago, Kyle Kingsbury, a well-known mixed martial arts guy, artist, and host of the *Kyle Kingsbury Podcast,* came to visit us. He had a toddler at the time. "You know, I just couldn't figure it out," he said. "I was lying in bed every night for nine and a half hours and still waking up every day feeling exhausted." But then Kyle got a watch that tracked his sleep and he realized that, because he had a little kid, he was waking up like thirty-five times a night—not because the toddler was rousing him all those times, but just in that nervous new parent, "Is my kid still alive?" kind of way. "Actually, it made me feel better," he said, "because I was finally able to make the connection."

Given that sleeping like a baby is mostly only possible if you actually *are* a baby (and sometimes not even then), we employ every possible strategy to ensure that we can get as much high-quantity, high-quality sleep as possible. Those strategies are what's known as "sleep hygiene"—a set of evidence-based behaviors that help ease the body and brain into a full and refreshing night's slumber. Most doctors will prescribe these best practices in lieu of sleeping pills for insomnia. We swear by them, are militant about adhering to them, and we think you will be, too, once you've worked them into your routine and seen what a difference a full night's sleep can make. These behaviors are your physical practice for Vital Sign 10. In this next section, we'll lay them out for you and explain why they're worthy of your devotion.

Physical Practice: A Better Shut-Eye Plan

Read any book on sleep, talk to any expert on slumber, and you'll learn the same important piece of information: Establishing a bedtime routine is paramount to successful sleeping. We can tell you this isn't just sleep-doctor-speak: Through personal experience we know that putting sleep hygiene practices in place night after night really works. Give your body the same cues repeatedly, and you'll find it easier to drift off and be more likely to sleep through the night. Here are the ten best practices we recommend for sleep hygiene.

1 GO TO SLEEP AND WAKE UP AT THE SAME TIME, EVEN ON WEEKENDS.

Just as if we were toddlers who need a strict sleep routine (at least that was how we rolled as parents), we try to go to bed at the same time every night and wake up at the same time every morning. The weekends might have a little more give, but not that much, and there's a reason for that. The sleep cycle likes habit. It will be easier to fall asleep at night and easier to wake up in the morning if you stay on the same schedule. Plus, you can't fully make up for lost weekday sleep by snoozing until noon on the weekend. Likewise, napping isn't a sound solution. Naps can be beneficial—if you sleep longer than thirty minutes, you may enter the restorative stage of deep sleep—but they can't make up for nighttime sleep deprivation. They can also make it harder to fall asleep, perpetuating the cycle. If you do nap, do it before 3 p.m.

2 MOVE THROUGHOUT YOUR DAY.

Presumably, if you're adhering to the various physical practices in this book, you're already doing this—particularly if you're walking à la Vital Sign 4. If you need a refresher on how walking relates to sleep, see page 111. (The short version: Walking fatigues the body and, if done during daylight, helps keep the circadian rhythm on track.) While we're on the subject of moving and sleep, we often get asked about whether it's okay to exercise at night. There is a plausible reason that this might be a bad idea. Exercise increases core temperature (more on this in a minute) and arousal in the body, which could make it harder to fall asleep. But there are so many variables, including how close to bedtime you exercise, whether your individual chronobiology makes you a night owl or morning person, and so on. What's most important about exercise is not when you do it but that you do it at all. Yes, if it's keeping you awake, try to adjust your schedule and bear in mind that morning cardiovascular exercise helps regulate the circadian rhythm. But don't automatically assume that exercising at night is a bad thing. As always, listen to your body.

3 BE CAREFUL WITH CAFFEINE.

Caffeine, whether you get it from coffee, tea, chocolate, energy drinks, or some other source (including decaffeinated drinks, which still have some caffeine), takes some time to be eliminated from the system—perhaps a lot more time than you were expecting. It takes four to six hours for half of the caffeine to be metabolized (different people metabolize it differently). And while its power to block sleep will be diminished once it's past its peak in the body, caffeine can still make it difficult to go to sleep hours later. One study found that people who had 400 milligrams of caffeine as far out as six hours before bed lost an average of one hour's sleep. That's about four eight-ounce cups of coffee—though caffeine counts vary by brewing method—or about one of Starbucks' oversized serving sizes. Since everyone is different, you'll need to establish your own caffeine cutoff time. Kelly's is 4 p.m., Juliet's is 2 p.m. Experiment to see what yours should be.

4 NO TECHNOLOGY IN THE ROOM; LIMIT IT BEFORE BEDTIME.

If you have a smartphone, this probably needs no explanation. Those little rectangular packets of news, gossip, connections to loved ones, work info, entertainment of every variety, calendars, health data, and so much more are truly hard to resist. They can keep you up to all hours scrolling, then "helpfully" wake you with

2 a.m. pings from your friend in London, and local news alerts. But that's just one part of it.

Throughout this book we've talked about how modern technology has moved us away from the behaviors our bodies are built for. We don't typically think of the lightbulb as modern technology—it's been around since the 1800s—but even this ubiquity of civilized life takes its toll on the body by artificially extending our day. You may remember that the release of melatonin, the spark that sets off sleepiness, is triggered by darkness. Artificial light delays the onset of melatonin and thus our natural sleepiness by hours. We're pretty used to that by now, establishing later bedtimes than our lightless forebears, but throw in some more contemporary lights—blue light–emitting LEDs that are today's norm—and you've upped the ante. Blue light, which has a more alerting effect than the light from incandescent bulbs, is what brightens TVs, game consoles, smartphones, tablets, and computers. You may be sitting in the dark, but the LED glow enveloping you is still sending a wake-up signal to your brain. Once you turn off all your devices, the alertness can linger, and as melatonin plays catchup, it can be a while before drowsiness sets in. Inevitably, this leads to less sleep overall and, research shows, less REM sleep in particular.

If you have an LED bulb in your bedside lamp, replacing it with an incandescent one to limit your exposure to blue light before bed is one step toward solving the problem. Banning technology from your bedroom and turning off technology altogether two to three hours before bedtime is also an ideal way to avoid its sleep-disturbing influence. We say "ideal" because we know that TV watching and the like are beloved evening activities. We're not saying not to do it at all, but now that you know the power of blue light to inhibit sleep, take stock of what's happening to you at night. Are you staying up too late and having trouble falling asleep when you finally do power off? Adjust your technology habits accordingly. For example: When we moved into our house, there was a television on the bedroom wall. We had never had a television in our bedroom before, so we were kind of excited. After about a month, when we found we were up late watching some show, we ripped it off the wall. It's been a technology-free space ever since.

But that's us. We know it's a lot to ask. At the very least, if you must have your phone on your nightstand, set it to "Do Not Disturb" during your sleep window. If you're not predisposed to get rid of your bedroom TV or give up watching it from the comfort of your bed, institute a curfew: It must go off at least a half hour before bedtime. Pick up a book till it's (incandescent) lights out.

5 DRINK VERY LITTLE ALCOHOL (OR NONE AT ALL).

Alcohol is a great con artist. It makes you believe it will help you sleep better, when in fact it is only setting you up for a night of tossing and turning. It's true that alcohol is a depressant and that it may in fact make you sleepy enough to nod off, but according to Berkeley's Matthew Walker, that's not really sleep. "The electrical brainwave state you enter via alcohol," he writes in *Why We Sleep*, "is not that of natural sleep; rather, it is akin to a light form of anesthesia." When sleep does set in, it's generally disrupted, and the otherwise elegantly timed sleep cycles are thrown into disarray. REM sleep, in particular, suffers, suppressed by chemicals released by the breakdown of alcohol in the system. The end result: Not good. Even relatively small amounts of alcohol quash the brain's ability to digest information.

Walker advises against drinking alcohol if you're after a good night's sleep. The Sleep Foundation advises imbibing no more than four hours before bedtime. Obviously, it's a personal choice, one you can make based on your goals. We're not teetotalers ourselves; we drink occasionally, mostly at celebratory times. We're persuaded, though, by the evidence showing that alcohol not only disturbs sleep, but—athletes beware—prevents some of the post-exercise tissue repair and regeneration that takes place during restorative sleep. By gathering the data of users of its wearable fitness tracker, the company WHOOP has been able to determine that heart rate variability and resting heart rate—measures of recovery and good health—are negatively affected when users report they've consumed alcohol the day before.

What's more, in a study the WHOOP people conducted with college athletes, they also found that those athletes who had as little as one drink sometimes took as long as four to five days to recover. Juliet has learned a lot from her own sleep tracker metrics. She hadn't had any alcohol for about five weeks and had just recovered from COVID when she went out with friends she hadn't seen for a long time. She had one drink. The next morning, her sleep tracker reported that she got a sleep quality score of 25 (out of 100). One drink had a more detrimental effect on her sleep than the virus did (that score was 32).

6 COOL DOWN.

Temperature is a key factor in helping set the wheels of the sleep machine in motion. One of the ways the circadian rhythm helps instigate sleep is by cooling your body down near bedtime. Along with the onset of darkness, this natural drop of about 2 to 3 degrees Fahrenheit in core temperature helps drive the release of melatonin. You can help this process along by keeping your bedroom temperature at 65 degrees—cool temps also aid in better sleep quality—and, though it may sound counterintuitive, by taking a warm bath or shower before bed. The warmth of the water draws blood to the surface of the skin and away from the center of the body, cooling the core. The relaxing effect of a bath or shower or a ten-minute dip in a hot tub if you've got one can also help ease your way into dreamland.

It would seem to make sense that a cold shower would modulate temperature and therefore enhance sleep as well, but studies testing out this supposition have had mixed results. In our personal sleep lab, we've found ice baths too close to bedtime fire us up (see A Study in Contrast: Hot and Cold Therapy, page 205), but we are not beyond using them to cool down pre-sleep when our un-air-conditioned home is steeped in peak summer heat.

7 WIND DOWN.

One of our friends, Kirk "Doc" Parsley, a physician and former Navy SEAL, recommends setting an alarm one hour before the time you plan to go to bed to give yourself time to prepare for sleep. This is the time to turn off devices (if you haven't already), switch to reading a book (the real kind), do some soft tissue mobilizations, take a warm bath or shower, and otherwise wind down from the day so you have an easier time falling asleep.

8 MAKE YOUR BEDROOM A DARK, QUIET PLACE.

If you are a light sleeper, meaning you wake up at the slightest creak or flash of a car headlight in the street, go for sensory deprivation. Blackout shades/curtains and earplugs are your friends.

9 OVERESTIMATE THE TIME YOU NEED TO SPEND IN BED.

In the Hours Count sleep assessment, we asked you to subtract time that you were in bed but not really asleep. One thing we learned from tracking our own sleep is that it's really common to have about an hour of wake time during what we assume is sleep.

That led to a big shift for us, realizing that if we actually wanted to get eight hours of sleep, we actually had to be lying in bed for nine hours. So when people say, "I went to bed at ten, woke up at six, that's eight hours of sleep," we say—not so fast. That was probably only seven hours of sleep.

10 MIMIC YOUR BEDTIME ROUTINE WHEN YOU TRAVEL.

Travel, especially when there's jet lag involved, can pose a challenge to sleep. Late-night business dinners, vacation activities, and so on throw a wrench into regular sleep schedules. Okay, understood. There are going to be nights where you can only sleep five hours, and there's no way around that. But you can limit the damage by doubling down on all the pro-sleep practices you do at home, including holding off on alcohol.

When we get to our destination, we don't go crazy trying to figure out where the gym is or where we can exercise (travel is hard enough on the body). We simply go for a walk to help tire ourselves out for sleep and, if we're dealing with a time zone deficiency, to get exposure to daylight so we get in tune with the local time. Then, when it's time to go to bed, even if it's later than usual, we follow our typical routine: blackout curtains closed, eye masks on and earplugs in, phones and other technology off. Our brains are conditioned to associate these things with sleep and, like Pavlov's dog, they obey.

A PEEK INTO OUR BEDROOM

As we've already confessed, we are a bit obsessed with sleep, so, as you might imagine, our bedroom reflects our enthusiasm. Let us paint you a picture. First there are the blackout shades, ensuring that no light seeps in through the windows. To further lie down in darkness, we wear eye masks. We've got earplugs, too. On some nights we tape our mouths shut, too. (Not shaping up to be the sexy description you were expecting, eh?)

And there's more. We each have our own climate-controlled environments. Kelly, who naturally runs hot, sleeps on a Chili pad, which has cold water running through it that keeps his temperature from rising. The pad will also automatically adjust as it gets closer to morning so he doesn't wake up feeling like an ice cube. Juliet, over on her side of the bed, has a weighted blanket with a thermoregulating device that keeps her from getting too cold or too hot. There are lots of sleep accessories like this on the market now (including smart mattresses), high-tech solutions that can remedy the typical marriage temperature-variation spat.

We're the first to admit this is a little over-the-top, but sleep is our priority. And you don't have to invest in a high-priced gadget to get your temperature or other factors under control. A small fan and a washcloth dipped in water, frozen, then draped over your torso (or tucked into your armpit) can go a long way toward helping you cool your body down for sleep. Sleep masks and earplugs are inexpensive. White noise machines aren't too costly, either, if you find you need soothing sounds to help you drift off. If there's any takeaway from our personal sleep cave, it is that your bedroom doesn't have to conform to traditional standards of design. Find the accoutrements that will enhance your sleep and put them in place.

MAKING IT ALL WORK

24-HOUR DUTY CYCLE AND 21-DAY BUILT TO MOVE CHALLENGE

I F YOU WERE born thousands of years ago, you'd have no need to ask the question "How can I fit in all the things I need to do for my body?" All of those things would have just been part of your natural day-to-day life. But, hey, it's the twenty-first century, so here we are, most of us leading busy lives and some of us not used to making time for self-care.

We call our approach to working it all in the 24-Hour Duty Cycle. The name alludes to the fact that caring for the machinery—our body—is all within the revolution of a full day. We have a schedule, and we keep to it—more loosely on some days and with allowances when things get crazy and there's no way to make everything work. But, in general, we find that having a set of routine behaviors during the day and evening allows us to stay on course.

Everyone is different. Night owls and larks, for instance, as we discussed in the previous chapter. Your day may not look like ours. *Ours* don't even look like ours, since we both approach the day a little differently. But a strategy that everyone can use is to look at your day and ask yourself, "What hours are within my control?" For most people, it's the hours on either side of 9 to 5 (give or take an hour or two for you over-achievers), plus maybe some time during lunch. Once you have your time frame, you can start slotting in the things you need to do.

We know that some of you will go through the book and create your own adventure, working the various physical practices into your day as it suits. But for those of you who like a formalized plan, we want to give you two things. One is an example of what a typical Built to Move day might look like—that's the 24-Hour Duty Cycle. The other is the 21-Day Built to Move Challenge.

Over the years, we've created many challenges for members of The Ready State, each one skewed to a different element of fitness (e.g., indoor cycling, squatting). The 21-Day Built to Move Challenge here is designed specifically as a road map to the mobilizations and other practices in this book. It will help you try out all the different ones, and determine which resonate, which should be your top priority, and which ones you may be able to do less often. It starts slow, having you take ten days to do the tests while also beginning to layer in certain everyday practices and mobiliza-tions at the same time. We always think of our challenges as a gateway to helping people incorporate new habits into their lives. This challenge is no different. You've read all about how to get a durable body, a body that allows you to do everything you want to do with vigor and without pain. Now it's time to mobilize—in every sense of the word!

24-HOUR DUTY CYCLE

TIME	ACTIVITY
6:00 AM	Wake up. Drink a big glass of water with a pinch of sea salt and lemon. Putter around, get kids' lunches ready.
6:30 AM	Warm up for exercise, incorporating some mobilizations and breathing exercises. Work out.
7:30 AM	End work out. See kids out the door. Do a few more mobilizations. Take a walk to cool down (3,000 steps).
8:00 AM	Eat breakfast (⅓ of produce and protein quota for the day) and have coffee. Prepare lunch to take to work. Get dressed for the day.
9:00 AM	Begin work, using standing desk practices. Make phone calls while walking (1,000–2,000 steps). Do some balance play when taking a work break.
12:00 PM	Lunch (⅓ of produce and protein quota for the day). Take a walk after eating (3,000 steps).
1:00 PM	Back to work, using standing desk practices. Caffeine cut-off time—no more coffee today.
5:00 PM	Off duty, heading home. Get in a last walk for the day (3,000 steps).
5:30 PM	Make dinner (⅓ of produce and protein quota for the day).
6:30 PM	Dinner with the family.
7:30 PM	Dishes washed, family time. Sit on the floor while watching TV and chilling.
8:30 PM	Technology off. Hot tub or warm shower. 10 minutes of soft-tissue mobilizations.
9:30 PM	In bed, reading.
10:00 PM	Lights out. Zzzzzz.
10:00-6:00	SLEEP

21-DAY BUILT TO MOVE CHALLENGE

	TEST	EVERYDAY PRACTICES	MOBILIZATIONS
Day 1	Sit-and-Rise Test	Try various ground-sitting positions (pp. 43–45): · Cross-Legged Sitting · 90/90 Sitting · Long Sitting · One-Leg-Up Sitting	Seated Hamstring Mobilization (p. 46) Hamstring Lockouts (p. 47) Hip Opener (p. 48) Elevated Pigeon (p. 48)
Day 2	Breath-Hold Test	· Practice nose-only breathing throughout the day · Sit on the floor in various positions · 2 Sit-Stands (p. 203) · Extra Credit: Tape your mouth closed	Morning Spin-Up (p. 71) Trunk Mobilization (p. 72) T-Spine Mobilization 1 (p. 72)
Day 3	Couch Test	· Sit on the floor in various positions · Practice nose-only breathing throughout the day · 3 Sit-Stands (p. 203)	Couch Stretch (p. 94) Quad-Thigh Mobilization (p. 96) Extra Credit: Kneeling/Standing/Couch Isometrics (pp. 97–99)
Day 4	Steps-Per-Day Inventory	· Sit on the floor in various positions · Walk 8–10K steps · Try barefoot walking · 4 Sit-Stands (p. 203) · Extra Credit: Rucking	Hamstring Lockouts (p. 47) Couch Stretch (p. 94) Elevated Pigeon (p. 48)
Day 5	Part 1: Airport Scanner Arms-Raise Test Part 2: Shoulder Rotation Test	· Sit on the floor in various positions · Walk 8–10K steps · Practice intentional walking · Practice nose-only breathing throughout the day · 5 Sit-Stands (p. 203)	Wall Hang (p. 144) T-Spine Mobilization 2 (p. 145) Rotator Cuff Mobilization (p. 146) Extra Credit: Try/practice Worm-Up push-up technique (p. 147)

	TEST	EVERYDAY PRACTICES	MOBILIZATIONS
Day 6	Part 1: 800-Gram Count Part 2: Protein Count	· Eat 800 grams fruits and vegetables · Consume individualized grams protein · Sit on the floor in various positions · Walk 8–10K steps (practice nose-only breathing while walking) · 6 Sit-Stands (p. 203) · Extra Credit: Barefoot walking or rucking	Seated Hamstring Mobilization (p. 46) Quad-Thigh Mobilization (p. 96)
Day 7	Squat Test	· Eat 800 grams fruits and vegetables · Consume individualized grams protein · Sit on the floor in various positions · Walk 8–10K steps (try three post-meal walks per day) · Practice nose-only breathing throughout the day · 7 Sit-Stands (p. 203)	Deep Squat Hang-Out (p. 204) Tabata Squats (p. 204)
Day 8	Part 1: SOLEC (Stand On One Leg, Eyes Closed) Test Part 2: Old Man Balance Test	· Eat 800 grams fruits and vegetables · Consume individualized grams protein · Sit on the floor in various positions · Walk 8–10K steps · Practice Y-Balance Mobilization (p. 222) · 8 Sit-Stands (p. 203) · Extra Credit: Jumping rope or bouncing	Bone Saw (p. 223) Calf Stretch Crossover (p. 224) Foot Play (p. 225)

	TEST	EVERYDAY PRACTICES	MOBILIZATIONS
Day 9	Sitting Inventory	· Eat 800 grams fruits and vegetables · Consume individualized grams protein · Sit on the floor in various positions · Walk 8–10K steps (intentional walking) · Practice balance play · Accumulate 30 minutes of standing while working or dynamic sitting · Practice nose-only breathing throughout the day · 9 Sit-Stands (p. 203) · Extra Credit: Rucking	Rotator Cuff Mobilization (p. 146) T-Spine Mobilization 1 (p. 72) Extra Credit: Try/practice Worm-Up push-up technique (p. 147)
Day 10	Part 1: Hours Count	· Eat 800 grams fruits and vegetables · Consume individualized grams protein · Sit on the floor in various positions · Walk 8–10K steps (practice nose-only breathing while walking) · Practice balance play · Follow sleep hygiene practices · Accumulate 40 minutes of standing while working or dynamic sitting · 10 Sit-Stands (p. 203)	Wall Hang (p. 144) Trunk Mobilization (p. 72)

	TEST	EVERYDAY PRACTICES	MOBILIZATIONS
Day 11		· Eat 800 grams fruits and vegetables · Consume individualized grams protein · Sit on the floor in various positions · Walk 8–10K steps (try three post-meal walks per day) · Practice Y-Balance Mobilization (p. 222) · Follow sleep hygiene practices · Accumulate 50 minutes of standing while working or dynamic sitting · 11 Sit-Stands (p. 203)	Seated Hamstring Mobilization (p. 46) Hamstring Lockouts (p. 47) Elevated Pigeon (p. 48)
Day 12		· Eat 800 grams fruits and vegetables · Consume individualized grams protein · Sit on the floor in various positions · Walk 8–10K steps (practice nose-only breathing while walking) · Practice Old Man Balance Test (p. 211) · Follow sleep hygiene practices · Accumulate 1 hour of standing while working or dynamic sitting · 12 Sit-Stands (p. 203)	Hip Opener (p. 48) Quad-Thigh Mobilization (p. 96)

	TEST	EVERYDAY PRACTICES	MOBILIZATIONS
Day 13		· Eat 800 grams fruits and vegetables · Consume individualized grams protein · Sit on the floor in various positions · Walk 8–10K steps (intentional walking) · Practice balance play · Follow sleep hygiene practices · Accumulate 1 hour and 10 minutes of standing while working or dynamic sitting · 13 Sit-Stands (p. 203)	Couch Stretch (p. 94) Deep Squat Hang-Out (p. 204) Elevated Pigeon (p. 48)
Day 14		· Eat 800 grams fruits and vegetables · Consume individualized grams protein · Sit on the floor in various positions · Walk 8–10K steps (practice nose-only breathing while walking) · Practice Y-Balance Mobilization (p. 222) · Follow sleep hygiene practices · Accumulate 1 hour and 20 minutes of standing while working or dynamic sitting · 14 Sit-Stands	Bone Saw (p. 223) Foot Play (p. 225) Calf Stretch Crossover (p. 224) Tabata Squats (p. 204)

	TEST	EVERYDAY PRACTICES	MOBILIZATIONS
Day 15		· Eat 800 grams fruits and vegetables · Consume individualized grams protein · Sit on the floor in various positions · Walk 8–10K steps (include some time barefoot walking) · Practice balance play · Follow sleep hygiene practices · Accumulate 1 hour and 30 minutes of standing while working or dynamic sitting · 15 Sit-Stands (p. 203)	T-Spine Mobilization 2 (p. 145) Wall Hang (p. 144) Extra Credit: Try/practice Worm-Up push-up technique (p. 147)
Day 16		· Eat 800 grams fruits and vegetables · Consume individualized grams protein · Sit on the floor in various positions · Walk 8–10K steps (practice nose-only breathing while walking) · Practice balance play · Follow sleep hygiene practices · Accumulate 1 hour and 40 minutes of standing while working or dynamic sitting · Extra Credit: Jumping rope or bouncing · 16 Sit-Stands (p. 203)	Hip Opener (p. 48) Kneeling/Standing/ Couch Isometrics (pp. 97–99)

	TEST	EVERYDAY PRACTICES	MOBILIZATIONS
Day 17		· Eat 800 grams fruits and vegetables · Consume individualized grams protein · Sit on the floor in various positions · Walk 8–10K steps (try three post-meal walks per day) · Practice Y-Balance Mobilization (p. 222) · Follow sleep hygiene practices · Accumulate 1 hour and 50 minutes of standing while working or dynamic sitting · Practice nose-only breathing at work · 17 Sit-Stands (p. 203)	Trunk Mobilization (p. 72) Quad-Thigh Mobilization (p. 96)
Day 18		· Eat 800 grams fruits and vegetables · Consume individualized grams protein · Sit on the floor in various positions · Walk 8–10K steps (intentional walking) · Practice Old Man Balance Test (p. 211) · Follow sleep hygiene practices · Accumulate 2 hours of standing while working or dynamic sitting · Practice nose-only breathing at work · 18 Sit-Stands (p. 203)	Couch Stretch (p. 94) Bone Saw (p. 223)

	TEST	EVERYDAY PRACTICES	MOBILIZATIONS
Day 19		· Eat 800 grams fruits and vegetables · Consume individualized grams protein · Sit on the floor in various positions · Walk 8–10K steps (intentional walking) · Follow sleep hygiene practices · Accumulate 2 hours and 10 minutes of standing while working or dynamic sitting · Practice nose-only breathing at work · 19 Sit-Stands (p. 203)	Seated Hamstring Mobilization (p. 46) Hamstring Lockouts (p. 47) Deep Squat Hang-Out (p. 204)
Day 20		· Eat 800 grams fruits and vegetables · Consume individualized grams protein · Sit on the floor in various positions · Walk 8–10K steps (intentional walking) · Practice balance play · Follow sleep hygiene practices · Accumulate 2 hours and 20 minutes of standing while working or dynamic sitting · Practice nose-only breathing at work · 20 Sit-Stands (p. 203)	Rotator Cuff Mobilization (p. 146) T-Spine Mobilizations 1 and 2 (pp. 72, 145) Extra Credit: Try/practice Worm-Up push-up technique (p. 147)

	TEST	EVERYDAY PRACTICES	MOBILIZATIONS
Day 21		· Eat 800 grams fruits and vegetables · Consume individualized grams protein · Sit on the floor in various positions · Walk 8–10K steps (intentional walking) · Practice nose-only breathing while walking · Practice Y-Balance Mobilization (p. 222) · Follow sleep hygiene practices · Accumulate 2 hours and 30 minutes of standing while working or dynamic sitting · Practice nose-only breathing at work · 21 Sit-Stands (p. 203) · Extra Credit: Rucking	Couch Stretch (p. 94) Deep Squat Hang-Out (p. 204) Tabata Squats (p. 204)

AFTERWORD

NEVER DO NOTHING: THE CASE FOR EXERCISE

F ROM ITS OPENING pages up until the page you are now reading, this book has not been about exercise—exercise, that is, in the sense of sustained cardiovascular workouts and/or a regular strength-training regimen. But we couldn't in good conscience close this book without advocating for both of the above forms of physical activity. While the ten Vital Signs in this book will help you develop and maintain a resilient and robust body, adding in regular exercise will take you to an even higher level of durability. Exercise is your supplemental insurance plan.

Many of you already work out often and enthusiastically, so we don't really have to make the case for exercise to you. And the truth is, if you're following the physical practices in this book—specifically the 8,000 to 10,000 steps protocol—then you *are* exercising to some degree. But wherever you are in the trajectory from non-exerciser to athlete, keep reading. We think that some of the things we've learned about fitness in both a professional and personal capacity can be of value.

The Built to Move Mindset

At this stage of the game, it's the rare person who doesn't know the health benefits of exerting oneself in the name of physical fitness. So we won't go on and on about the lowered risk of heart disease, diabetes, some cancers, depression, obesity, and more. You've heard it all; you know exercise is the best type of preventive medicine available. Millions claim it makes them feel great, too, and we'd have to agree.

Less clear-cut is how much exercise you should be doing, what kind, when, where, with whom, and so on. The recommendations shift, but here are the most recent *Physical Activity Guidelines for Americans,* as issued by the U.S. Department of Health and Human Services: Adults should get at least 150 minutes of moderate-intensity aerobic physical activity or 75 minutes of vigorous-intensity physical activity, or an equivalent combination, each week. Adults should also do muscle-strengthening activities of moderate or greater intensity and that involve all major muscle groups on two or more days a week. If everyone followed these guidelines (and the ten physical practices in this book), we could change the world. But we also know that life's ebbs and flows can cause good intentions to crumble like a cookie underfoot. That's why we add another exercise principle to the list of guidelines: Always Do Something—or, as Dave Spitz likes to spin it, Never Do Nothing.

Dave Spitz is a former college track-and-field athlete who was humming along as an investment banker when he decided to give it up and train for the 2008 Olympic trials as a weightlifter. While his Olympic dream fell short, he has since opened a well-regarded training facility and is a sought-after coach. One of the things Dave told us when we interviewed him for our podcast was that he'd like to disabuse people of the notion that gym owners work out all the time. (As former Cross-Fit gym owners ourselves, we knew exactly what he was talking about.) With a business to run, employees to manage, and three kids in the mix, he doesn't have enough hours in the day to exercise as much as he'd like to. So instead of torturing himself over what he can't do, Dave adopted the motto "Never Do Nothing." Every day he makes sure that he gets in at least 10,000 steps, has a good night's sleep, and eats some vegetables. Then he trains when he can.

Dave's maxim perfectly expresses how we feel about exercise. We are all for routines—just look at our 24-Hour Duty Cycle (page 267)—and heartily agree with the *Physical Activity Guidelines for Americans.* But when you believe that you must fulfill a particular regimen and something gets in the way, it's tempting—no, *common*—to do nothing at all. If your boss keeps you after hours and you miss your Pilates class, you shrug it off, go home, and watch TV. You have a late night and don't have the energy to get up and meet your mountain biking group in the morning, so you think, "Well, my exercise opportunity for the day is shot." It is not. Go for a walk. Do some mobility and balance exercises. Jump rope for ten minutes. Don't let perfect be the enemy of good. Your body wants to—needs to—move, and in that regard any activity is good. Do what you can, but don't do nothing.

When our children were very young and demanding of our time, we were also growing two businesses. It was all we could do to get a protein bar down, let alone set aside time to lift a barbell. So Kelly developed something he called "the 10s." At 10 p.m. each night, when things had quieted down, we'd do 10 pull-ups, 10 push-ups, and 10 squats on repeat for 10 minutes. That was our exercise for the day. It wasn't high caliber, but it helped us retain our strength and kept us fit enough so that when we did resume some of our sports and gym activities, we were still in decent shape. And yet that was really the least of it. What we were doing during those ten minutes each night was training for the demanding work- and child-centric life we were living. Training not just to train, but training for life.

Becoming an Active Person

At its simplest, exercise is something to do to make your life better. And for the most part, it doesn't matter how you do it. If we have one specific recommendation, it would be to do some strength training. As a culture we seem to have more easily embraced cardio activities like running and cycling and hiking, but there's a lag in adopting strengthening exercises. And it doesn't take much. Get a kettlebell and lift it every day, graduating to a heavier one when it gets easy. Do one push-up daily and build on it. Ruck (page 123). Walk up hills.

Science tells us that, due to genetics, different people respond differently to exercise. Some people get more of a dopamine (pleasure chemical) hit from activity; some have less tolerance for the discomfort it causes. So if you avoid exercise, there may in fact be a biological reason. You might have to try a little harder than some to pick up that kettlebell or do that push-up or walk that hill or push the pedals on a bike or swim that lap or hit that tennis ball or jog around the block or do Pilates or join a tai chi class or experiment with Zumba or paddle a kayak or stream a Peloton session or shoot hoops or swing a golf club or pick up pickleball . . . Do you see what we're getting at? There are so many ways to exercise; there is something for everyone. Experiment so you can find what you like to do (or can at least tolerate). The idea is just to move your body because, as you know by now, your body is built to move!

We have created a library of free follow-along content and resources to support your Built to Move journey. Just scan the code below for more.

SCAN ME

ACKNOWLEDGMENTS

Two people are at the top of the long list of people who made *Built to Move* possible. The first is our agent, Dado Derviskadic, who patiently waited for us for many years to be at the right place and in the right frame of mind to write this book. His vision, wisdom, guidance, and creative brilliance throughout have blown our minds and bound him to us for the rest of our book-writing lives. Thank you, Dado. You are stuck with us.

The second is our cowriter, Daryn Eller, without whom this book would not exist. Daryn took our (often) frenetic energy and excitement about this topic and somehow managed to transform it into a relatable, accessible, and eminently readable book. It is also very difficult to write a book in two authors' voices and she managed that task with perfection by honoring both of our perspectives and contributions. Daryn's willingness to be the test subject for all of the Vital Signs and her advice about what would and wouldn't work for our readers has been invaluable and made this book what it is today. Daryn, your next-level writing chops, professionalism, and kindness have made this experience a joy from start to finish. We hope this is the first of many times we get to work with you. Thank you.

We'd also like to thank our editor, Andrew Miller, for his attention to detail, keen insight, and willingness to be a test subject for the Vital Signs to bring his unique perspective to the book. Josh McKible, the human body is the most complex structure in the known universe. Thank you for your amazing illustrations that help make the invisible visible in this book. We still can't believe our good fortune in being able to work with the team of true experts on our greater Knopf team, including Chris Gillespie, Emily Reardon, Sara Eagle, Matthew Sciarappa, and Tiara Sharma.

Special thank-you to Reagan Arthur for believing in us and our vision for this book and for supporting us fully. We are truly humbled and honored to be writing a book under the Knopf banner. Tim O'Connell, thank you for your early support and advocacy for this book.

This book would also not have been possible without the support of our entire Ready State team, including Margaret Garvey, Lisa Schwartz, Dave Beatie, Nicole Jerner, Ben Hardy, Ryan Fredericks, Mike Sloat, Chris Jerard, Kaitlin Lyons, and Sean Greenspan and his team. If you are reading this, it's because of their day-to-day hard work in supporting The Ready State brand and helping us get the word out on our website, on social media, and beyond about this book. They take care of so many details, small and large, that are never seen or acknowledged by the greater community. We are amazed every day by what we can pull off as much as we do with a small and mighty team. We see you and thank you.

Georgia and Caroline. We are so proud of the mature and capable young women you have both become. Georgia, thank you for being so damn kind and competent. What other sixteen-year-old kid cooks healthy dinners from scratch for the whole family on the regular? Caroline, thank you for making us laugh and reminding us there is so much joy to be experienced every day in life. This book is dedicated to you both because, if we've done one thing right as parents, it's taught you that you have to keep moving.

Thank you to the brilliant EC Synkowski for allowing us to feature the #800gChallenge in this book. It's such a simple yet brilliant idea that could not be more essential in a world with ever changing and confusing messages about what we should and should not eat.

To Gabby Reece and Laird Hamilton for your friendship and support of us, always.

Joyce Shulman, thank you for cutting through the noise in the health and fitness space to say that people need to move more and connect with one another more and that walking is the perfect way to do that.

Stacy Sims, we are so lucky to have connected with you all those years ago. We have relied on you for so much advice over the years and consider you a friend and mentor. Thank you for your willingness to support us and answer our questions, even from halfway across the world in New Zealand.

To the original built-to-movers, Janet and Warren Wiscombe, Juliet's parents, and their respective spouses, Ed Lai and Helenka Wiscombe. You'll never see a healthier group of seventy-plus-year-olds. We learned by their example starting in childhood that simple health habits (many of which are in this book), applied consistently, are the way to keep moving well into your seventies and beyond. Thank you also to each one of them for helping us raise our awesome kids so that we could manage to be parents and also have an expansive professional life.

Thank you to Wes Kitts, Dave Spitz, Chris Hinshaw, Mark Bell, Jesse Burdick, Stan Efferding, Joe DeFranco, Travis Mash, Mike Burgener, Gray Cook, and Chris Duffin for your stories, tests, anecdotes, and inspiration for this book.

To Kelly's parents, Don and Hallie Ward, who have been showing up to races and events all over the planet for as long as Kelly can remember. Don's view as a DO and Hallie's perspective as a psych professor were the original influence on body and mind for Kelly. All you need to do is show up at their home in the Colorado mountains to be reminded that we all need more fresh air and our own skulk of foxes. They've also had a sauna longer than anyone else in our lives.

To Juliet's brother, Tom Wiscombe, and his partner, Marrikka Trotter. We aren't sure how we all ended up choosing the entrepreneur path in life, but it's been extra special to be on a parallel journey with you. Thank you for your counsel, support, and commiseration, and of course for insisting that our first book be called *Becoming a Supple Leopard*.

We also won the lottery of friendship in life and we'd like to thank the following people for loving on us in this life (in no particular order because they are all awesome), for being test dummies for all our wacky health ideas, and for sticking by us as friends even though our schedule is not often conducive to hanging out as much as we'd like: Soman Chainani, Jim + Tricia Lesser, Erin Cafaro, Tim Ferriss, Bill Owens, Matt Vincent, Rich Froning, Jason Khalipa, Margaret Garvey, Mike Norman, Lisa + Zach Schwartz, Beth Dorsey + Jeff Trauba, Darcy Gomez + Chris Young, Adrienne Graf + Adam Forest, Diana Kapp + David Singer, Robin + Chris Donohoe, Brody Reiman + Serge Gerlach, Ben + Ariel Zvaifler, Jameson + Elena Garvey, Alice Tacheny + Michael Lynn, Orea Roussis, Anastacia + Steve Maggioncalda, Heidi Taglio + Michael Hazelrigg, Pam + Bernard Lauper, Kelli + Brendan Robertson, Kristina + John Doxon, Mitra + CJ Martin, Matt and Tezza Hermann, Allison + TJ Belger, Leigh + Thad Reichley, Justin + Clea Hovey, Levi Leipheimer, Shane Sigle, Jami Tikkanen, John Welbourn, Jen Widerstrom, Rachel Balkovec, Stuart McMillan, Caity + Bill Henniger, Kyla Channell and Sid Jamotte, Dan Zmolik + Maria Quiroga, Rebecca Rusch, Julie Munger + Abigail Polsby, Beth Rypins, Sue Norman, Damara Stone, Anik + Jay Wild, Kenny Kane, Marc Goddard, Travis Jewett, Kingsley Yew, Danny Matta, Sean McBride, Sue Wyatt, Erica Providenza, Catherine + JD Cafaro, Diane Fu, Mark Anderson, Jamie + Mary Collie, Christina and Eron Kosmowski, Stacy + Matthew Perry, Noel Kosiek, Cody West + Maija Blaufuss, Emma Bird, Chris Gustavson, Catherine Picard, Carolin Loose, Corby + Molly Leith, Gretchen Weber + TJ Murphy, Rich + Wendy Starrett, Cindy + Phil Rach, Natasha Wiscombe, Kristina Lai + Justine Okello, Lauren + Andy Lai, Kate Courtney, and Rory McKernan.

Lastly, thank you to our Ready State partners, whose products and support have helped us stay healthy, recover from one too many surgeries, and have all the right tools to play hard: Chad Nelson at YETI, Jeff Byers at Momentous, Ryan Duey + Michael Garrett at Plunge, Mike Sinyard at Specialized, Ryan Heaney at Marc Pro, Star Sage at Hyperice, Craig Storey and Jason McCann at Vari, and Todd Youngblood at Chili Sleep.

SOURCES

INTRODUCTION

"Chronic Back Pain." Health Policy Institute, Georgetown University. https://hpi
.georgetown.edu/backpain.
"Obesity and Overweight." National Center for Health Statistics, Centers for Disease
Control and Prevention. www.cdc.gov/nchs/fastats/obesity-overweight.htm.
"Wellness Industry Statistics and Facts." Global Wellness Institute. https://
globalwellnessinstitute.org/press-room/statistics-and-facts.

VITAL SIGN 1: GETTING UP AND DOWN OFF THE FLOOR

Adolph, Karen E., Whitney G. Cole, Meghana Komati, et al. "How Do You Learn to
Walk? Thousands of Steps and Dozens of Falls per Day." *Psychological Science* 23,
no. 11 (2012): 1387–94. DOI: 10.1177/0956797612446346.
Attia, Peter. "Fasting, Metformin, Athletic Performance, and More." *Tim Ferriss
Show*, podcast episode #398, November 27, 2019. https://tim.blog/guest/peter
-attia/.
Barbosa Barreto de Brito, Leonardo, Ricardo Rabelo, Sardinha Djalma, et al.
"Ability to Sit and Rise from the Floor as a Predictor of All-Cause Mortality."
European Journal of Preventive Cardiology 21, no. 7 (July 2014): 892–98.
DOI: 10.1177/2047487312471759.
Cranz, Galen. *The Chair: Rethinking Culture, Body, and Design.* New York:
W. W. Norton, 1998.
Hewes, Gordon W. "World Distribution of Certain Postural Habits." *American
Anthropologist* 57, no. 2 (1955): 231–44.
Lieberman, Daniel. *Exercised: The Science of Physical Activity, Rest and Health.*
London: Penguin, 2021.

"Breathing into a Paper Bag Can Calm Anxiety Attack." Ask the Doctors, UCLA
Health, September 16, 2021. https://connect.uclahealth.org.

Chalaye, Philippe, Philippe Goffaux, Sylvie Lafrenaye, and Serge Marchand.
"Respiratory Effects on Experimental Heat Pain and Cardiac Activity."
Pain Medicine 10, no. 8 (November/December 2009): 1334–40. DOI:
10.1111/j.1526-4637.2009.00681.x.

Dallam, George, Steve McClaran, Daniel Cox, and Carol Foust. "Effect of Nasal
Versus Oral Breathing on VO2max and Physiological Economy in Recreational
Runners Following an Extended Period Spent Using Nasally Restricted Breathing."
International Journal of Kinesiology and Sports Science 6, no. 2 (April 2018):
22–29. DOI: 10.7575/aiac.ijkss.v.6n.2p.22.

Flanell, Michael. "Lifetime Effects of Mouth Breathing." *Orthodontic Practice US,*
July 30, 2020. https://orthopracticeus.com.

Hudson, Daisy-May. "Inside the Superhuman World of Wim Hof: The Iceman." *Vice,*
video, 39:39, 2015. https://video.vice.com.

Learn, Joshua Rapp. "Science Explains How the Iceman Resists Extreme Cold."
Smithsonian Magazine, May 22, 2018.

Lundberg, J. O. N., G. Settergren, S. Gelinder, et al. "Inhalation of Nasally Derived
Nitric Oxide Modulates Pulmonary Function in Humans." *Acta Physiologica
Scandinavica* 158, no. 4 (December 1996): 343–47. DOI: 10.1046/j.1365-201X
.1996.557321000.x.

McKeown, Patrick. "Comparing the Oxygen Advantage® and Wim Hof Methods."
Oxygen Advantage. Accessed August 27, 2021. https://oxygenadvantage.com
/wim-hof.

Mummolo, Stefano., A. Nota, S. Caruso, et al. "Salivary Markers and Microbial Flora
in Mouth Breathing Late Adolescents." *BioMed Research International* 8687608
(2018). DOI: 10.1155/2018/8687608.

Nestor, James. *Breath: The New Science of a Lost Art.* New York: Riverhead, 2020.

O'Hehir, Trisha, and Amy Francis. "Mouth vs. Nasal Breathing." *Dentaltown
Magazine,* September 2012. www.dentaltown.com.

Schünemann H. J., J. Dorn, B. J. Grant, et al. "Pulmonary Function Is a Long-Term
Predictor of Mortality in the General Population: 29-Year Follow-Up of the Buffalo
Health Study." *Chest* 118, no. 3 (September 2000): 656–64. DOI: 10.1378
/chest.118.3.656.

Stephen, Michael J. *Breath Taking: The Power, Fragility, and Future of Our
Extraordinary Lungs.* New York: Atlantic Monthly Press, 2021. See pp. 19–23.

Templer, Paul. "Experience: I Was Swallowed by a Hippo." *Guardian,* May 4, 2013.

Templer, Paul. "Hippo Attack Survivor Paul Templer." *Verbal Shenanigans,* podcast episode #43, April 2, 2015. https://verbalshenaniganspodcast.podbean.com.

VITAL SIGN 3: EXTEND YOUR HIPS

Lehecka, Bryan J., Jessica Turley, Aaron Stapleton, et al. "The Effects of Gluteal Squeezes Compared to Bilateral Bridges on Gluteal Strength, Power, Endurance, and Girth." *PeerJ* 7 (2019): e7287. DOI: 10.7717/peerj.7287.

VITAL SIGN 4: WALK THIS WAY

Bassett, David R., Holly R. Wyatt, Helen Thompson, et al. "Pedometer-Measured Physical Activity and Health Behaviors in U.S. Adults." *Medicine and Science in Sports and Exercise* 42, no. 10 (October 2010): 1819–25. DOI: 10.1249/MSS .0b013e3181dc2e54.

Buman, Matthew P., and Abby C. King. "Exercise as a Treatment to Enhance Sleep." *American Journal of Lifestyle Medicine* 4, no. 6 (2010): 500–14. DOI: 10.1177/1559827610375532.

Carter, Sophie, Richard Draijer, Sophie Holder, et al. "Regular Walking Breaks Prevent the Decline in Cerebral Blood Flow Associated with Prolonged Sitting." *Journal of Applied Physiology* 125, no. 3 (2018): 790–98. DOI: 10.1152 /japplphysiol.00310.2018.

Dall, Philippa Margaret, Sarah Lesley Helen Ellis, Brian Martin Ellis, et al. "The Influence of Dog Ownership on Objective Measures of Free-Living Physical Activity and Sedentary Behaviour in Community-Dwelling Older Adults: A Longitudinal Case-Controlled Study." *BMC Public Health* 17, no. 1 (2017): 496. DOI: 10.1186/s12889-017-4422-5.

DiSalvo, David. "Using a Standing Desk Could Give Your Brain a Boost." *Forbes,* January 18, 2016.

Ekelund, Ulf, Jakob Tarp, Morten Fagerland, et al. "Joint Associations of Accelerometer-Measured Physical Activity and Sedentary Time with All-Cause Mortality: A Harmonised Meta-Analysis in More Than 44,000 Middle-Aged and Older Individuals." *British Journal of Sports Medicine* 54 (December 2020): 1499–1506. DOI: 10.1136/bjsports-2020-103270.

GORUCK. "About GORUCK." www.goruck.com.

Heesch, Kristiann C., Yolanda R. van Gellecum, Nicola W. Burton, et al. "Physical Activity, Walking, and Quality of Life in Women with Depressive Symptoms."

American Journal of Preventive Medicine 48, no. 3 (March 2015): 281–91. DOI: 10.1016/j.amepre.2014.09.030.

Jayedi, Ahmad, Ali Gohari, and Sakineh Shab-Bidar. "Daily Step Count and All-Cause Mortality: A Dose-Response Meta-Analysis of Prospective Cohort Studies." *Sports Medicine* 52, no. 1 (2022): 89–99. DOI: 10.1007/s40279-021-01536-4.

McDowell, C. P., B. R. Gordon, K. L. Andrews, et al. "Associations of Physical Activity with Anxiety Symptoms and Status: Results from the Irish Longitudinal Study on Ageing." *Epidemiology and Psychiatric Sciences* 28, no. 4 (2019): 436–45. DOI: 10.1017/S204579601800001X.

Neighmond, Patti. "Exercising to Ease Pain: Taking Brisk Walks Can Help." NPR, September 23, 2019. www.npr.org.

Neumann, Janice. "Regular Walking Can Help Ease Depression." Reuters Health, January 30, 2015.

O'Keefe, Evan L., and Carl J. Lavie. "A Hunter-Gatherer Exercise Prescription to Optimize Health and Well-Being in the Modern World." *Journal of Science in Sport and Exercise* 3 (2021): 147–57. DOI: 10.1007/s42978-020-00091-0.

Oppezzo, Marily, and Daniel L Schwartz. "Give Your Ideas Some Legs: The Positive Effect of Walking on Creative Thinking." *Journal of Experimental Psychology: Learning, Memory, and Cognition* 40, no. 4 (2014): 1142–1152.

Patel, Alpa V., Leslie Bernstein, Anusila Deka, et al. "Leisure Time Spent Sitting in Relation to Total Mortality in a Prospective Cohort of US Adults." *American Journal of Epidemiology* 172, no. 4 (August 2010): 419–29. DOI: 10.1093/aje/kwq155.

Polaski, Anna M., Amy L. Phelps, Kimberly A. Szucs, et al. "The Dosing of Aerobic Exercise Therapy on Experimentally-Induced Pain in Healthy Female Participants." *Scientific Reports* 9 (2019): 14842. DOI: 10.1038/s41598-019-51247-0.

Ratey, John. "Why Walking Matters." *Here & Now*, WBUR (Boston), May 19, 2014. www.wbur.org/hereandnow/2014/05/19/why-walking-matters.

Ratey, John. "Exercise Is the Best Medicine for Our Brain." Center for Discovery, YouTube video, 32:59, October 24, 2017. www.youtube.com/watch?v=oTUPSUIAw1c.

"Staying Active." The Nutrition Source, Harvard School of Public Health. www.hsph.harvard.edu/nutritionsource/staying-active.

Stillman, Jessica. "A Neuroscientist Explains Exactly How Awesome Exercise Is for Your Brain." *Inc.*, June 22, 2021. www.inc.com.

Sullivan Bisson, Alycia N., Stephanie A. Robinson, and Margie E. Lachman. "Walk to a Better Night of Sleep: Testing the Relationship Between Physical Activity and Sleep." *Sleep Health* 5, no. 5 (October 2019): 487–94. DOI: 10.1016/j.sleh.2019.06.003.

Uchida, Sunao, Kohei Shioda, Yuko Morita, et al. "Exercise Effects on Sleep Physiology." *Frontiers in Neurology* 3 (April 2012): 48. DOI: 10.3389/fneur .2012.00048.

U.S. Department of Health and Human Services. *Physical Activity and Health: A Report of the Surgeon General.* Atlanta: Centers for Disease Control and Prevention, 1996. www.cdc.gov/nccdphp/sgr/index.htm.

van Uffelen, Jannique G. Z., Yolanda R. van Gellecum, Nicola W. Burton, et al. "Sitting-Time, Physical Activity, and Depressive Symptoms in Mid-Aged Women." *American Journal of Preventive Medicine* 45, no. 3 (September 2013): 276–81. DOI: 10.1016/j.amepre.2013.04.009.

Wang, Feifei, and Szilvia Boros. "Effects of a Pedometer-Based Walking Intervention on Young Adults' Sleep Quality, Stress and Life Satisfaction: Randomized Controlled Trial." *Journal of Bodywork and Movement Therapies* 24, no 4 (October 2020): 286–92. DOI: 10.1016/j.jbmt.2020.07.011.

Wayman, Erin. "Becoming Human: The Evolution of Walking Upright." *Smithsonian Magazine,* August 6, 2012.

VITAL SIGN 5: FUTURE-PROOF YOUR NECK AND SHOULDERS

Andersen, Lars L., Michael Kjær, Karen Søgaard, et al. "Effect of Two Contrasting Types of Physical Exercise on Chronic Neck Muscle Pain." *Arthritis & Rheumatology* 59, no. 1 (January 2008): 84–91. DOI: 10.1002/art.23256.

DocMorris. "Take Care of Yourself. Doc Morris Christmas Advert 2020." YouTube video, 2:55, December 21, 2020. www.youtube.com/watch?v=-BDq6BQXOWs.

Mortensen, Peter, Anders I. Larsen, Mette K. Zebis, et al. "Lasting Effects of Workplace Strength Training for Neck/Shoulder/Arm Pain Among Laboratory Technicians: Natural Experiment with 3-Year Follow-Up." *Biomed Research International* (2014): 845851. DOI: 10.1155/2014/845851.

VITAL SIGN 6: EAT LIKE YOU'RE GOING TO LIVE FOREVER

"About SWAN." SWAN: Study of Women's Health Across the Nation. www.swan study.org/about/about-swan.

Aune, Dagfinn, Edward Giovannucci, Paolo Boffetta, et al. "Fruit and Vegetable Intake and the Risk of Cardiovascular Disease, Total Cancer and All-Cause Mortality: A Systematic Review and Dose-Response Meta-Analysis of Prospective Studies." *International Journal of Epidemiology* 46, no. 3 (June 2017): 1029–56. DOI: 10.1093/ije/dyw319.

Babault, Nicolas, Christos Païzis, Gaëlle Deley, et al. "Pea Proteins Oral Supplementation Promotes Muscle Thickness Gains During Resistance Training: A Double-Blind, Randomized, Placebo-Controlled Clinical Trial vs. Whey Protein." *Journal of the International Society of Sports Nutrition* 12 (2015): 3. DOI: 10.1186/s12970-014-0064-5.

Banaszek, Amy, Jeremy R. Townsend, David Bender, et al. "The Effects of Whey vs. Pea Protein on Physical Adaptations Following 8-Weeks of High-Intensity Functional Training (HIFT): A Pilot Study." *Sports* 7, no. 1 (2019): 12. DOI: 10.3390/sports7010012.

Baum, Jamie I., Il-Young Kim, and Robert R. Wolfe. "Protein Consumption and the Elderly: What Is the Optimal Level of Intake?" *Nutrients* 8, no. 6 (June 2016): 359. DOI: 10.3390/nu8060359.

Carbone, John W., and Stefan M. Pasiakos. "Dietary Protein and Muscle Mass: Translating Science to Application and Health Benefit." *Nutrients* 11, no. 5 (May 2019): 1136. DOI: 10.3390/nu11051136.

"Diabetes Statistics." National Institute of Diabetes and Digestive and Kidney Diseases. www.niddk.nih.gov/health-information/health-statistics/diabetes -statistics.

"Diet Review: Intermittent Fasting for Weight Loss." The Nutrition Source, Harvard School of Public Health. www.hsph.harvard.edu/nutritionsource/healthy-weight /diet-reviews/intermittent-fasting.

Drew, Liam. "Fighting the Inevitability of Ageing." *Nature Outlook* 555 (March 7, 2018). DOI: 10.1038/d41586-018-02479-z.

Easter, Michael. *The Comfort Crisis: Embrace Discomfort to Reclaim Your Wild, Happy, Healthy Self.* New York: Rodale, 2021.

García-Esquinas, Esther, Berna Rahi, Karine Peres, et al. "Consumption of Fruit and Vegetables and Risk of Frailty: A Dose-Response Analysis of 3 Prospective Cohorts of Community-Dwelling Older Adults." *American Journal of Clinical Nutrition* 104, no. 1 (July 2016): 132–42. DOI: 10.3945/ajcn.115.125781.

Gorissen, Stefan H. M., Julie J. R. Crombag, Joan M. G. Senden, et al. "Protein Content and Amino Acid Composition of Commercially Available Plant-Based Protein Isolates." *Amino Acids* 50, no. 12 (2018): 1685–1695.

Kojima, Narumi, Miji Kim, Kyoko Saito, et al. "Lifestyle-Related Factors Contributing to Decline in Knee Extension Strength Among Elderly Women: A Cross-Sectional and Longitudinal Cohort Study." *PloS ONE* 10, no. 7 (2015): e0132523. DOI: 10.1371/journal.pone.0132523.

Kolata, Gina. "In a Yearlong Study, Scientists Find No Benefit to Time-Restricted Eating." *New York Times,* April 20, 2022.

Liu, Deying, Yan Huang, Chensihan Huang, et al. "Calorie Restriction With or

Without Time-Restricted Eating in Weight Loss." *New England Journal of Medicine* 386, no. 16 (April 2022): 1495–1504. DOI: 10.1056/NEJMoa2114833.

Lowe, Dylan A., Nancy Wu, Linnea Rohdin-Bibby, et al. "Effects of Time-Restricted Eating on Weight Loss and Other Metabolic Parameters in Women and Men with Overweight and Obesity: The TREAT Randomized Clinical Trial." *JAMA Internal Medicine* 180, no. 11 (2020): 1491–99. DOI: 10.1001/jamainternmed.2020.4153.

McCall, Pete. "9 Things to Know About How the Body Uses Protein to Repair Muscle Tissue." ACE, March 5, 2018. www.acefitness.org/education-and-resources /professional/expert-articles/6960.

Meroño, Tomás, Raúl Zamora-Ros, Nicole Hidalgo-Liberona, et al. "Animal Protein Intake Is Inversely Associated with Mortality in Older Adults: The InCHIANTI Study." *Journals of Gerontology (Series A): Medical Sciences* 20, no. 20 (2022): glab334. DOI: 10.1093/gerona/glab334.

"Micronutrients for Health." Micronutrient Information Center, Linus Pauling Institute, Oregon State University. https://lpi.oregonstate.edu/mic.

Morell, P., and S. Fiszman. "Revisiting the Role of Protein-Induced Satiation and Satiety." *Food Hydrocolloids* 68 (July 2017): 199–210. DOI: 10.1016/j.foodhyd .2016.08.003.

Neacsu, Madalina, Claire Fyfe, Graham Horgan, and Alexandra M. Johnstone. "Appetite Control and Biomarkers of Satiety with Vegetarian (Soy) and Meat-Based High-Protein Diets for Weight Loss in Obese Men: A Randomized Crossover Trial." *American Journal of Clinical Nutrition* 100, no. 2 (August 2014): 548–58. DOI: 10.3945/ajcn.113.077503.

"Preserve Your Muscle Mass." Harvard Health Publishing, February 19, 2016. www .health.harvard.edu/staying-healthy/preserve-your-muscle-mass.

Putra, Christianto, Nicolai Konow, Matthew Gage, et al. "Protein Source and Muscle Health in Older Adults: A Literature Review." *Nutrients* 13, no. 3 (February 2021): 743. DOI: 10.3390/nu13030743.

Synkowski, EC. "The 800gChallenge." Optimize Me Nutrition. https://optimize menutrition.com/800g.

Tomey, Kristin M., MaryFran R. Sowers, Carolyn Crandall, et al. "Dietary Intake Related to Prevalent Functional Limitations in Midlife Women." *American Journal of Epidemiology* 167, no. 8 (April 2008): 935–43. DOI: 10.1093/aje /kwm397.

Webb, Densie. "Protein for Fitness: Age Demands Greater Protein Needs." *Today's Dietitian* 17, no. 4 (April 2015): 16. www.todaysdietitian.com.

Dubois, Blaise, and Jean-Francois Esculier. "Soft-Tissue Injuries Simply Need PEACE and LOVE." *British Journal of Sports Medicine* 54, no. 2 (2020): 72–73.

Kawashima, Masato, Noriaki Kawanishi, Takaki Tominaga, et al. "Icing after Eccentric Contraction-Induced Muscle Damage Perturbs the Disappearance of Necrotic Muscle Fibers and Phenotypic Dynamics of Macrophages in Mice." *Journal of Applied Physiology* (1985) 130, no. 5 (2021): 1410–1420.

St. Sauver, Jennifer L., David O. Warner, Barbara P. Yawn, et al. "Why Patients Visit Their Doctors: Assessing the Most Prevalent Conditions in a Defined American Population." *Mayo Clinic Proceedings* 88, no. 1 (2013): 56–67.

VITAL SIGN 7: SQUAT!

Bhattacharya, Sudip, Vijay Chattu, and Amarjeet Singh. "Health Promotion and Prevention of Bowel Disorders Through Toilet Designs: A Myth or Reality?" *Journal of Education and Health Promotion* 8 (2019): 40. DOI: 10.4103/jehp .jehp_198_18.

Hof, Wim. "Cold Therapy." Wim Hof Method. www.wimhofmethod.com/cold -therapy.

Hof, Wim. *The Wim Hof Method: Activate Your Full Human Potential.* Boulder, CO: Sounds True, 2020.

Laukkanen, Jari A., Tanjaniina Laukkanen, and Setor K. Kunutsor. "Cardiovascular and Other Health Benefits of Sauna Bathing: A Review of the Evidence." *Mayo Clinic Proceedings* 93, no. 8 (August 2018): 1111–21. DOI: 10.1016/j.mayocp .2018.04.008.

Machado, Aryane Flauzino, Paulo Henrique Ferreira, Jéssica Kirsch Micheletti, et al. "Can Water Temperature and Immersion Time Influence the Effect of Cold Water Immersion on Muscle Soreness? A Systematic Review and Meta-Analysis." *Sports Medicine* 46, no. 4 (April 2016): 503–14. DOI: 10.1007/s40279-015-0431-7.

Nevitt, Michael C., Ling Xu, Yuqing Zhang, et al. "Very Low Prevalence of Hip Osteoarthritis Among Chinese Elderly in Beijing, China, Compared with Whites in the United States: The Beijing Osteoarthritis Study." *Arthritis and Rheumatism* 46, no. 7 (July 2002): 1773–79. DOI: 10.1002/art.10332.

Zhang, Sarah. "Why Can't Everyone Do the 'Asian Squat'?" *Atlantic*, March 16, 2018.

Cho, HyeYoung, Michel J. H. Heijnen, Bruce A. Craig, and Shirley Rietdyk. "Falls in Young Adults: The Effect of Sex, Physical Activity, and Prescription Medications." *PloS ONE* 16, no. 4 (2021): e0250360. DOI: 10.1371/journal.pone.0250360.

Colledge, N. R., P. Cantley, I. Peaston, et al. "Ageing and Balance: The Measurement of Spontaneous Sway by Posturography." *Gerontology* 40, no. 5 (1994): 273–78. DOI: 10.1159/000213596.

El-Khoury, Fabienne, Bernard Cassou, Marie-Aline Charles, and Patricia Dargent-Molina. "The Effect of Fall Prevention Exercise Programmes on Fall Induced Injuries in Community Dwelling Older Adults: Systematic Review and Meta-Analysis of Randomised Controlled Trials." *BMJ* 347, no. 7934 (2013): f6234. DOI: 10.1136/bmj.f6234.

Ferlinc, Ana, Ester Fabiani, Tomaz Velnar, and Lidija Gradisnik. "The Importance and Role of Proprioception in the Elderly: A Short Review." *Materia Socio-Medica* 31, no. 3 (September 2019): 219–21. DOI: 10.5455/msm.2019.31.219-221.

Hrysomallis, Con. "Relationship Between Balance Ability, Training and Sports Injury Risk." *Sports Medicine* 37, no. 6 (2007): 547–56. DOI: 10.2165/00007256-200737 060-00007.

James, Melissa K., Mauricia C. Victor, Syed M. Saghir, and Patricia A. Gentile. "Characterization of Fall Patients: Does Age Matter?" *Journal of Safety Research* 64 (February 2018): 83–92. DOI: 10.1016/j.jsr.2017.12.010.

"Keep on Your Feet—Preventing Older Adult Falls." Injury Center, Centers for Disease Control and Prevention. www.cdc.gov/injury/features/older-adult-falls.

Myers, Dan. "This 'Die Hard' Relaxation Hack Is Actually Brilliant." *Active Times,* July 17, 2018. www.theactivetimes.com.

Petrella, R. J., P. J. Lattanzio, and M. G. Nelson. "Effect of Age and Activity on Knee Joint Proprioception." *American Journal of Physical Medicine & Rehabilitation* 76, no. 3 (May 1997): 235–41. DOI: 10.1097/00002060-199705000-00015.

Ribeiro, Fernando, and José Oliveira. "Aging Effects on Joint Proprioception: The Role of Physical Activity in Proprioception Preservation." *European Review of Aging and Physical Activity* 4 (2007): 71–76. DOI: 10.1007/s11556-007-0026-x.

Sherrington, Catherine, Nicola Fairhall, Wing Kwok, et al. "Evidence on Physical Activity and Falls Prevention for People Aged 65+ Years: Systematic Review to Inform the WHO Guidelines on Physical Activity and Sedentary Behaviour." *International Journal of Behavioral Nutrition and Physical Activity* 17 (2020): 144. DOI: 10.1186/s12966-020-01041-3.

Tsang, William W. N., and Christina W. Y. Hui-Chan. "Effects of Tai Chi on Joint Proprioception and Stability Limits in Elderly Subjects." *Medicine and Science*

in Sports and Exercise 35, no. 12 (December 2003): 1962–71. DOI: 10.1249/01
.MSS.0000099110.17311.A2.

Tucker, Larry A., J. Eric Strong, James D. LeCheminant, and Bruce W. Bailey. "Effect
of Two Jumping Programs on Hip Bone Mineral Density in Premenopausal
Women: A Randomized Controlled Trial." *American Journal of Health Promotion*
29, no. 3 (January 2015): 158–64. DOI: 10.4278/ajhp.130430-QUAN-200.

Weiss, Audrey J., Lawrence D. Reid, and Marguerite L. Barrett. "Overview of
Emergency Department Visits Related to Injuries, by Cause of Injury, 2017."
Statistical Brief #266, Healthcare Cost and Utilization Project, Agency for
Healthcare Research and Quality, U.S. Department of Health and Human
Services, November 2020. www.hcup-us.ahrq.gov.

VITAL SIGN 9: CREATE A MOVEMENT-RICH ENVIRONMENT

Agarwal, Shuchi, Craig Steinmaus, and Carisa Harris-Adamson. "Sit-Stand
Workstations and Impact on Low Back Discomfort: A Systematic Review and
Meta-Analysis." *Ergonomics* 61, no. 4 (2018): 538–52. DOI: 10.1080/00140139
.2017.1402960.

"Americans Sit Almost 10 Hours a Day (On Average)." Get America Standing.
https://getamericastanding.org.

Blake, Jamilia J., Mark E. Benden, and Monica L. Wendel. "Using Stand/Sit
Workstations in Classrooms: Lessons Learned from a Pilot Study in Texas."
Journal of Public Health Management and Practice 18, no. 5 (September/October
2012): 412–15. DOI: 10.1097/PHH.0b013e3182215048.

Bontrup, Carolin, William R. Taylor, Michael Fliesser, et al. "Low Back Pain and Its
Relationship with Sitting Behaviour Among Sedentary Office Workers." *Applied
Ergonomics* 81 (2019): 102894. DOI: 10.1016/j.apergo.2019.102894.

Crespo, Noe C., Sarah L. Mullane, Zachary S. Zeigler, et al. "Effects of Standing and
Light-Intensity Walking and Cycling on 24-h Glucose." *Medicine and Science in
Sports and Exercise* 48, no. 12 (December 2016): 2503–11. DOI: 10.1249/MSS
.0000000000001062.

Dornhecker, Marianela, Jamilia J. Blake, Mark Benden, et al. "The Effect of Stand-
Biased Desks on Academic Engagement: An Exploratory Study." *International
Journal of Health Promotion and Education* 53, no. 5 (April 2015): 271–80. DOI:
10.1080/14635240.2015.1029641.

Dunstan, David W., Shilpa Dogra, Sophie E. Carter, and Neville Owen. "Sit Less and
Move More for Cardiovascular Health: Emerging Insights and Opportunities."
Nature Reviews Cardiology 18 (September 2021): 637–48. DOI: 10.1038/s41569
-021-00547-y.

Garrett, Gregory, Mark Benden, Ranjana Mehta, et al. "Call Center Productivity Over 6 Months Following a Standing Desk Intervention." *IIE Transactions on Occupational Ergonomics and Human Factors* 4, no. 2–3 (2016): 188–95. DOI: 10.1080/21577323.2016.1183534.

Harrell, Eben. "How 1% Performance Improvements Led to Olympic Gold." *Harvard Business Review*, October 30, 2015.

Koepp, Gabriel A., Graham K. Moore, and James A. Levine. "Chair-Based Fidgeting and Energy Expenditure." *BMJ Open Sport & Exercise Medicine* 2, no. 1 (2016): e000152–e000152.

Levine, James A. *Get Up! Why Your Chair Is Killing You and What You Can Do About It*. New York: Palgrave Macmillan, 2014.

Levine, James A., Sara J. Schleusner, and Michael D. Jensen. "Energy Expenditure of Nonexercise Activity." *American Journal of Clinical Nutrition* 72, no. 6 (December 2000): 1451–54. DOI: 10.1093/ajcn/72.6.1451.

Ma, Jiameng, Dongmei Ma, Zhi Li, and Hyunshik Kim. "Effects of a Workplace Sit-Stand Desk Intervention on Health and Productivity." *International Journal of Environmental Research and Public Health* 18 (2021): 11604. DOI: 10.3390/ijerph182111604.

Mehta, Ranjana K., Ashley E. Shortz, Mark E. Benden. "Standing Up for Learning: A Pilot Investigation on the Neurocognitive Benefits of Stand-Biased School Desks." *International Journal of Environmental Research and Public Health* 13 (2015): 0059. DOI: 10.3390/ijerph13010059.

Shive, Holly. "Standing Desks—From Bright Idea to Successful Business Venture." *Vital Record*, Texas A&M Health, January 21, 2014. https://vitalrecord.tamhsc.edu.

Swartz, Ann M., Nathan R. Tokarek, Scott J. Strath, et al. "Attentiveness and Fidgeting While Using a Stand-Biased Desk in Elementary School Children." *International Journal of Environmental Research and Public Health* 17 (2020): 3976. DOI: 10.3390/ijerph17113976.

Ussery, Emily N., Geoffrey P. Whitfield, Janet E. Fulton, et al. "Trends in Self-Reported Sitting Time by Physical Activity Levels Among US Adults, NHANES 2007/2008–2017/2018." *Journal of Physical Activity and Health* 18 (2021): S74–S83. DOI: 10.1123/jpah.2021-0221.

Vlahos, James. "Is Sitting a Lethal Activity?" *New York Times*, April 14, 2011.

Wick, Katharina, Oliver Faude, Susanne Manes, et al. "I Can Stand Learning: A Controlled Pilot Intervention Study on the Effects of Increased Standing Time on Cognitive Function in Primary School Children." *International Journal of Environmental Research and Public Health* 15 (2018): 356. DOI: 10.3390/ijerph15020356.

Winkler, Elisabeth A. H., Sebastien Chastin, Elizabeth G. Eakin, et al. "Cardiometabolic Impact of Changing Sitting, Standing, and Stepping in the

Workplace." *Medicine and Science in Sports and Exercise* 50, no. 3 (March 2018): 516–24. DOI: 10.1249/MSS.0000000000001453.

Zeigler, Zachary S., Sarah L. Mullane, Noe C. Crespo, et al. "Effects of Standing and Light-Intensity Activity on Ambulatory Blood Pressure." *Medicine and Science in Sports and Exercise* 48, no. 2 (February2016): 175–81. DOI: 10.1249/MSS.0000000000000754.

VITAL SIGN 10: UNLEASH YOUR SUPERPOWER: SLEEP

Baker, Peter. "The Mellowing of William Jefferson Clinton." *New York Times Magazine,* May 26, 2009.

Carey, Benedict. "Why It Hurts to Lose Sleep." *New York Times,* January 28, 2019.

Chattu, Vijay Kumar, Dilshad Manzar, Soosanna Kumary, et al. "The Global Problem of Insufficient Sleep and Its Serious Public Health Implications." *Healthcare* 7, no. 1 (2019): 1. DOI: 10.3390/healthcare7010001.

Chaput, Jean-Philippe, Jean-Pierre Després, Claude Bouchard, et al. "Short Sleep Duration Is Associated with Reduced Leptin Levels and Increased Adiposity: Results from the Québec Family Study." *Obesity* 15, no. 1 (2007): 253–261.

Cohen, Sheldon, William J. Doyle, Cuneyt M. Alper, et al. "Sleep Habits and Susceptibility to the Common Cold." *Archives of Internal Medicine* 169, no. 1 (2009): 62–67. DOI: 10.1001/archinternmed.2008.505.

Drake, Christopher, Timothy Roehrs, John Shambroom, and Thomas Roth. "Caffeine Effects on Sleep Taken 0, 3, or 6 Hours Before Going to Bed." *Journal of Clinical Sleep Medicine* 9, no. 11 (November 2013): 1195–1200. DOI: 10.5664/jcsm.3170.

Fenton, S., T. L. Burrows, J. A. Skinner, and M. J. Duncan. "The Influence of Sleep Health on Dietary Intake: A Systematic Review and Meta-Analysis of Intervention Studies." *Journal of Human Nutrition and Dietetics* 34, no. 2 (April 2021): 273–85. DOI: 10.1111/jhn.12813.

Hafner, Marco, Martin Stepanek, Jirka Taylor, et al. "Why Sleep Matters—The Economic Costs of Insufficient Sleep: A Cross-Country Comparative Analysis." *Rand Health Quarterly* 6, no. 4 (2017): 11.

Hanlon, Erin C., Esra Tasali, Rachel Leproult, et al. "Sleep Restriction Enhances the Daily Rhythm of Circulating Levels of Endocannabinoid 2-Arachidonoylglycerol." *Sleep* 39, no. 3 (March 2016): 653–64. DOI: 10.5665/sleep.5546.

Huang, Baozhen, Yanlin Niu, Weiguo Zhao, et al. "Reduced Sleep in the Week Prior to Diagnosis of COVID-19 Is Associated with the Severity of COVID-19." *Nature and Science of Sleep* 12 (2020): 999–1007. DOI: 10.2147/NSS.S263488.

Krause, Adam J., Aric A. Prather, Tor D. Wager, et al. "The Pain of Sleep Loss:

A Brain Characterization in Humans." *Journal of Neuroscience* 39, no. 12 (March 2019): 2291–2300. DOI: 10.1523/JNEUROSCI.2408-18.2018.

Leary, Eileen B., Kathleen T. Watson, Sonia Ancoli-Israel, et al. "Association of Rapid Eye Movement Sleep with Mortality in Middle-Aged and Older Adults." *JAMA Neurology* 77, no. 10 (2020): 1241–51. DOI: 10.1001/jamaneurol.2020.2108.

Pacheco, Danielle. "Sleep and Blood Glucose Levels." Sleep Foundation, April 21, 2022. www.sleepfoundation.org/physical-health/sleep-and-blood-glucose-levels.

Prather, Aric A., Denise Janicki-Deverts, Martica H. Hall, and Sheldon Cohen. "Behaviorally Assessed Sleep and Susceptibility to the Common Cold." *Sleep* 38, no. 9 (September 2015): 1353–59. DOI: 10.5665/sleep.4968.

Spaeth, Andrea M., David F. Dinges, and Namni Goel. "Effects of Experimental Sleep Restriction on Weight Gain, Caloric Intake, and Meal Timing in Healthy Adults." *Sleep* 36, no. 7 (July 2013): 981–90. DOI: 10.5665/sleep.2792.

St. Hilaire, Melissa A., Melanie Rüger, Federico Fratelli, et al. "Modeling Neurocognitive Decline and Recovery During Repeated Cycles of Extended Sleep and Chronic Sleep Deficiency." *Sleep* 40, no. 1 (January 2017). DOI: 10.1093/sleep/zsw009.

Suni, Eric. "How Sleep Deprivation Affects Your Heart." Sleep Foundation, April 1, 2022. www.sleepfoundation.org/sleep-deprivation/how-sleep-deprivation-affects-your-heart.

Suni, Eric. "Melatonin and Sleep." Sleep Foundation, April 8, 2022. www.sleepfoundation.org/melatonin.

Suni, Eric. "Sleep Statistics." Sleep Foundation, May 13, 2022. www.sleepfoundation.org/how-sleep-works/sleep-facts-statistics.

Van Deusen, Mark. "Physiological Effects of Alcohol Through the Lens of WHOOP." WHOOP, October 16, 2020. www.whoop.com/thelocker/alcohol-affects-body-hrv-sleep.

AFTERWORD: NEVER DO NOTHING

American Physiological Society (APS). "Hate Exercise? It May Be in Your Genes." ScienceDaily, November 4, 2016. www.sciencedaily.com.

U.S. Department of Health and Human Services. *Physical Activity Guidelines for Americans.* 2nd ed. Washington, D.C.: U.S. Department of Health and Human Services, 2018, p. 8. https://health.gov/sites/default/files/2019-09/Physical_Activity_Guidelines_2nd_edition.pdf

"Walking: Why Walk? Why Not!" Physical Activity Initiatives, Centers for Disease Control and Prevention. www.cdc.gov/physicalactivity/walking.

INDEX

hip extension and, 91
mobilizations and, 20, 45
pain and, 67–70
sleep and, 251–52
walking and, 103, 113–15, *115*
brain-derived neurotrophic factor
  (BDNF), 114
brain.fn app, 255
Brandeis University, 112
BRCA genes, 137
breast cancer, 137–39
breastfeeding, 152, 153
breath, getting out of, 55
Breath-Hold Test, 54–56, 59, *270*
breathing (Vital Sign 2), 15, 23, 25, 52–75
  apps to aid, 74–75
  assessment
    Breath-Hold Test, 54–56, 59, 61, *270*
  conscious, 52, 69
  Core by Hyperice, 75
  Couch Stretch and, 95
  Couch Test and, 79
  dynamic sitting and, 244
  as intensity gauge, 25
  mobilizations, 52, 70–75
    Morning Spin-Up, 71
    Trunk Mobilization, 72, *72*
    T-Spine Mobilization 1, 72–73, *73*
    Tape Your Mouth Closed, 73–74
    Wim Hof Method and, 69
  nose vs. mouth, 63–66
  nose-only, 53, *270–72, 276–78*
  slower, 53, 63, 66
  pain and, 67–70, 129
  positioning and, 61–63
  roadmap to better, 56–57
  shoulder-neck problems and, 139–40
  stability and energy and, 58–59
  surgery and, 139

underwater challenge, 60–61
walking and, 108–9
Breath (Nestor), 64, 73
Brillat-Savarin, Jean Anthelme, 149
British Cycling, 234
British Journal of Sports Medicine, 192
bronchial tubes, 56, 64
Built to Move plan, 6–8, 16
  defining terms, 19–23
  equipment for, 27
  how to use, 16–19
  making it all work, 14, 267–78
  mindset and, 280–81
  questions about, 23–27
  things to know before beginning, 27–28
Bulgarian Split Squat, 99, *99*
butt squeezes, 86–87

caffeine, 9, 163, 254, 256, 260
calcium, 179
Calf Stretch Crossover, 224, *224, 271, 274*
calming, 66, 72, 112–13
calories, 106–7, 122–23, 151, 153, 180,
  183, 232, 234–35, 237, 253
calves, 42, *44,* 122
cancer, 103, 168
capillaries, 56
car, backing up, 144
carbohydrates, 154
carbon dioxide (CO$_2$) tolerance, 53–55,
  57, 59–61, 66, 75, 123
cardiovascular system, 57, 66, 103, 111,
  122–23, 168, 170, 205, 246
carotenoids, 154
cartilage, 109, 172
casein, 175, 176
Centenarian Olympics, 88–89
Centers for Disease Control and
  Prevention (CDC), 12, 208, 248

Italy, 170
Iyengar, B.K.S., 70

Japan, 3, 36, 129, 233
jaw, 64
Jobs, Steve, 12
joints, 11–12, 19–21, 23–24, 109–10, 133, 187
jumping, 221, 223–24
jumping rope, 201, 221, 223, *271, 275*

Karnazes, Dean, 161
Keto diet, 151
kettlebells, 125, 130, 282
Kingsbury, Kyle, 258
Kipchoge, Eliud, 64
kitchen scale, 156
Kitts, Wes, 58
Kneeling Isometric, 97–98, *97,* 245, *270, 275*
kneeling on floor, 40
knee pain, 78, 109, 187, 189
knees, 38, 84–86, 91, 194, 199–200
knee surgery, 150, 155
Kobe University, 191
Korea, 36

lactose intolerance, 176
Lamaze method, 68
legs
    One-Leg-Up Sitting, 45, *45, 270*
    Seated Hamstring and, 45
    Sit-and-Rise Test and, 30
    SOLEC (Stand On One Leg Eyes Closed), 209–11, *210,* 214, *271*
legumes, 159, 160, *182*
Leonardo da Vinci, 214
leptin, 253
Levine, James, 232

Licht, Bob, 218
Lieberman, Daniel, 39
ligaments, 110, 172
lighting, bedroom, 261, 266
Liverpool John Moores University, 113
loading, 22, 38
loneliness, 118
Long Sitting 42, 44, *44, 270*
low back, *43,* 78, 84–86, 190, 194
lumbar spine, 194
lunges, 78
lungs, 56, 66
lymphatic system, 38, 110–11, 191, 205
Maastricht University, 176
macronutrients, 154
magnesium, 179
marathon runners, 64, 68, 129, 161
Mash, Travis, 92
mastectomy, double, 137–38
Mayo Clinic, 187, 232
Mayweather, Floyd, 64
McCarthy, Emily, 125
McCarthy, Jason, 125
McGregor, Conor, 64
McKeown, Patrick, 54
meat, 151, 159–60, 170, *181*
meditation, 40, 66, 71
Mediterranean diet, 151
melatonin, 256, 261, 263
meniscus transplant surgery, 150
menopause, 221
mental focus, 69–70
metabolic flexibility, 161–67
metabolism, 102, 185
Micronesia, 36
micronutrients, 7, 15, 151–58, 162, 167–69
minerals, 154, 167
Mirkin, Gabe, 191

neck and shoulders (Vital Sign 5) *(continued)*
  importance and basic workings of, 127–30, 140–41
  mobilizations, 143–48, 201
    Push-Ups, 147–48, *148*
    Rotator Cuff Mobilization, 146, *146*
    Shoulder Flexion Mobilization, 143
    T-Spine Mobilization 1, *73*
    T-Spine Mobilization 2, 145, *145*
    Wall Hang, 144, *144*
    Worm Push-Up, 148, *148*
  resolving conundrum of, 139–43
  surgery and, 137–39
neck pain, 53–54, 66, 129, 141, 142
nervous system, 21, 70, 154
Nestor, James, 64, 66, 73–74
neurotransmitters, 113–14, 253
New England Journal of Medicine, 185
New York Times, 232
New Zealand, 3
Next Level (Sims), 221
night sweats, 186
90/90 sitting, 42, 44, *44, 270*
99 Walks, 116, 118
nitric oxide (NO), 65–66
normal accident theory, 17
nose breathing, 53, 63–66, *271*
Nose-Breathing Walk, 73, 119, 123, *274*
NREM (non-rapid eye movement) sleep, 257
NSAIDs, 188
nuts and seeds, 159, 180

obesity, 103, 182
Obesity Solutions Initiative, 232
Old Man Balance Test, 211–12, *211, 271, 273, 276*
Olympic Club, 34–35, 41

Olympics, 10, 25, 58, 129, 142, 234, 280
One-Leg-Up Sitting, 45, *45, 270*
osteoporosis, 103, 154
Oura, 249
oxygen intake, 53–54, 56–57, 66

paddling, 3–5, 67–68, 89–90, 135, 201, 218, 229, 282
pain, 186–92
  breathing and, 53, 54, 67–70, 109
  contract-and-relax and, 22
  First Aid Kit, 188
  healthcare provider and, 186–87
  hip extension and, 77
  icing and, 190–92
  long-duration sitting and, 189–90
  mobilizations and, 15, 24–25
  PEACE & LOVE protocol and, 192
  referred, 189
  RICE protocol and, 191–92
  self-soothing and, 190
  upstream-downstream thinking and, 188–89
  walking and, 109, 115
pain medication, 188
Paleo diet, 11, 151
pancreas, 162–63, *163*
panic attacks, 57
parasympathetic system, 26, 66, 69, 72
Parsley, Kirk "Doc," 264
pectorals, 138, 140
pedometers, 104, 105
Peloton bike, 11, 63, 90, 160
pelvic floor, 85, 122
pelvis, 37, 38, 40, 85–86
Phelps, Michael, 235
phenolic acids, 154
Physical Activity Guidelines for Americans, 280, 281

A NOTE ABOUT THE AUTHORS

Kelly Starrett, DPT, is a physical therapist and coauthor of the *New York Times* best sellers *Becoming a Supple Leopard* and *Ready to Run* and the *Wall Street Journal* best seller *Deskbound.* He is also the cofounder of The Ready State, which has revolutionized the field of movement health, mobility, and performance therapy. He consults with athletes and coaches from the NFL, NBA, NHL, MLB, the U.S. Olympic Team, Premier Rugby, Premier Soccer, and all branches of the U.S. elite armed forces, as well as with corporations on employee health and well-being. He lives in California.

Juliet Starrett, JD, is an entrepreneur, attorney, author, and podcaster. She is the cofounder and CEO of The Ready State, and the cofounder and chair of the board of StandUp Kids, a nonprofit dedicated to combating kids' sedentary lifestyles. She is coauthor of the *Wall Street Journal* best seller *Deskbound,* and was a professional whitewater paddler in a former life, winning three world championships and five national titles. She lives in California.

A NOTE ON THE TYPE

The text in this book was set in Miller, a transitional-style typeface designed by Matthew Carter (b. 1937) with assistance from Tobias Frere-Jones and Cyrus Highsmith of the Font Bureau. Modeled on the roman family of fonts popularized by Scottish type foundries in the nineteenth century, Miller is named for William Miller, founder of the Miller & Richard foundry of Edinburgh.

COMPOSED BY NORTH MARKET STREET GRAPHICS, LANCASTER, PENNSYLVANIA

PRINTED AND BOUND BY LAKESIDE BOOK COMPANY, CRAWFORDSVILLE, INDIANA

DESIGNED BY MAGGIE HINDERS